INTELLECTUAL DISABILITY IN THE TWENTIETH CENTURY

Transnational Perspectives on People, Policy and Practice

Edited by
Jan Walmsley and Simon Jarrett

First published in Great Britain in 2019 by

Policy Press
University of Bristol
1-9 Old Park Hill
Bristol
BS2 8BB
UK
t: +44 (0)117 954 5940
pp-info@bristol.ac.uk
www.policypress.co.uk

North America office:
Policy Press
c/o The University of Chicago Press
1427 East 60th Street
Chicago, IL 60637, USA
t: +1 773 702 7700
f: +1 773-702-9756
sales@press.uchicago.edu
www.press.uchicago.edu

© Policy Press 2019

British Library Cataloguing in Publication Data
A catalogue record for this book is available from the British Library

Library of Congress Cataloging-in-Publication Data
A catalog record for this book has been requested

978-1-4473-4457-5 hardback
978-1-4473-4458-2 ePdf
978-1-4473-4460-5 ePub
978-1-4473-4461-2 Mobi

Cover design by Robin Hawes
Front cover image: istock
Printed and bound in Great Britain by CPI Group (UK) Ltd,
Croydon, CR0 4YY
Policy Press uses environmentally responsible print partners

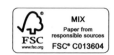

Contents

Notes on editors and contributors

Jan Walmsley is Visiting Chair, History of Learning Disabilities, Open University, UK. Jan is best known for two things: pioneering the study of the recent history of learning disability in the UK, particularly using oral and life history methods; and 'inclusive research' with people with learning disabilities. She is now an independent researcher, specialising in projects relating to learning disability history and co-produced research.

Simon Jarrett is an Associate Lecturer in History at Birkbeck, University of London, who has written widely on the history of intellectual disability. His areas of research include the transition from community to asylum over the eighteenth and nineteenth centuries and the impact of psychology after Darwin on the idea of 'idiocy'. He is editor of *Community Living* magazine, the UK's only print magazine about intellectual disability.

Jane Abraham has worked for over 25 years as a self-advocacy supporter and trainer in the UK, including with Mencap to devise and run Speaking Up training, and partnering with self-advocates to research and deliver awareness and social history training in schools. She spent 2016 in Accra, Ghana, where she volunteered with Inclusion Ghana and now splits her time between London and Accra.

Tobias Buchner currently holds a position as Senior Lecturer at the Department of Education, University of Vienna. His main research interests are inclusive education, learning biographies and inclusive research. Buchner is member of the Austrian Monitoring Board of the UNCRPD (United Nations Convention on the Rights of Persons with Disabilities), being responsible for science and research.

Yueh-Ching Chou is Professor of the Institute of Health and Welfare Policy, National Yang-Ming University, Taipei, Taiwan. Having a background in working with residents with an intellectual disability and their families in an institution, her research work and involvement in the deinstitutionalisation movement has aimed to promote independent living for disabled people in Taiwan.

Dr **Philip Ferguson** is Professor Emeritus at Chapman University in Orange, California. For over three decades he has pursued an interest in the field of disability studies, emphasising issues affecting people with intellectual disabilities. His research has focused on family/professional interactions, social policy and the history of intellectual disability.

Carol Hamilton's interest in institutionalisation comes from having worked with learning disabled people who had lived in institutional settings as young people, and with disability support staff who provided services to people who had come out of institutions. She is now Senior Lecturer in Disability and Inclusion Studies at University of Waikato in Hamilton, New Zealand and continues to ensure that this difficult aspect of New Zealand social history is not forgotten.

Danae Karydaki is a 20th-century historian interested in history of psychoanalysis, social history of psychiatry, gender history, and history of violence. She received her PhD from Birkbeck, University of London, and her current post-doctoral research on the Leros Psychiatric Hospital is funded by the Research Centre for the Humanities in Athens, Greece.

Dr **Gertraud Kremsner** studied inclusive education at the University of Vienna. Her dissertation, based on inclusive research together with six persons with learning difficulties, focused on experiences in (total) institutions. Gertraud Kremsner currently holds a post-doctoral research and senior lecturer position at the Center for Teacher Education (research group: inclusive education) at the University of Vienna.

Dr **Oliver Koenig** holds a post-doctoral position at the Department of Education at the University of Vienna. His current areas of teaching and research are: inclusive research, person–centred planning, and the intersections of transformative learning and organisational development in services for people with disabilities.

Lee-Ann Monk is a research associate in the Department of Archaeology and History, La Trobe University, Australia. Researching the history of Kew Cottages sparked her interest in the history of intellectual disability. She has since explored several aspects of that history, including sexuality and people with intellectual disability, and the exploitation of resident labour in institutions.

Monika Mužáková is Senior Lecturer at the Charles University in Prague, Faculty of Education, Department of Special Education. Prior to her academic career, Monika worked at the Czech Ministry of Health, where she was responsible for government subsidies to support non-governmental organisations of people with disabilities. Her ongoing research interests include history of special education and institutional care for people with disabilities. She has published two monographs in this area (*The history of association of the blind* in 2004, and *The experiences of parents of children with intellectual disabilities in Communist Czechoslovakia* in 2016). Monika's further research interests include parents with intellectual disabilities, and the impact of caregivers' long-term care for a family member with a disability or in palliative care. She has published 15 research articles in this area.

Auberon Jaleel Odoom is a Registered Organisation Development Practitioner and the National Co-ordinator of Inclusion Ghana. He is on the Council of Inclusion International and is currently the Board Chair of Inclusion Africa. He is also a board member of Special Olympics Ghana, the Autism Society of West Africa, the Ghana Federation of Disability Organisations, and the Africa Platform for Social Protection.

Guðrún V. Stefánsdóttir is Professor in Disability Studies at the University of Iceland, School of Education. Her research can be divided into three main research areas: first, life-history work and inclusive methodology; secondly, research on autonomy and people with intellectual disabilities; and thirdly, research projects concerning university education for people with intellectual disabilities.

Iva Strnadová is Associate Professor at the School of Education, University of New South Wales, Australia. Since 2005, Iva has conducted in more than 20 different research projects at national and international levels. She has published two books in the field of special education and disability studies, co-authored nine other books, and co-edited two books. Prior to her academic career, Iva worked for seven years with adults with intellectual disabilities and with autism. Her research aims to contribute to better understanding and the improvement of life experiences of people with disabilities. Her ongoing research interests include transitions in lives of people with disabilities, across the lifespan experiences of families caring for a child with a disability, women with intellectual disabilities, the well-being of people with intellectual disabilities and autism, inclusive education and ageing with intellectual disabilities.

Ágnes Turnpenny, PhD, works as a research associate at the Tizard Centre, University of Kent, UK. She is originally from Hungary, where she has done extensive research in social care institutions. Her research interests include well-being and social inclusion of people with intellectual disabilities.

Phyllis King Shui Wong is Assistant Professor in the Department of Social Work at The Chinese University of Hong Kong. Her current research work focuses on the self-determination, personal well-being, life planning and positive behavioural support of people with intellectual disabilities. For years, she has worked together with self-help groups and been involved in advocacy work to fight for the rights and better lives of people with disabilities in Hong Kong.

Introduction

Why this book, why now?

Thank you for coming to read this book. We believe it is the first of its kind to take a historical view of policy and practice in intellectual disability across continents, and we are certain it is unique in its emphasis on the impact on individuals. We are extremely proud of it and excited about its potential; however, it is not the book we intended to write.

The book started in early 2017 when Jan, one of the editors, approached Policy Press to enquire whether they would publish a book on the twentieth-century history of intellectual disability in England. The response was cautious – will it have an international element? I had been here before. The book I co-edited with John Welshman on the history of community care for people with intellectual disabilities (Welshman and Walmsley, 2006) had four international chapters, but the bulk was about the UK. This time, I (Jan) decided to go the whole hog, to attempt a transnational history, without in any way privileging the UK. I invited Simon to join me, and he accepted. And so the book began.

The book has chapters about 12 countries: six in Europe, one in North America, one in Africa, two in Asia and two in Australasia. We were deliberately not prescriptive when we invited authors to contribute. There are many reasonable ways to construct a century of a nation's history and we left it to chapter authors to choose their path rather than trying to impose uniformity. It means the chapters are all quite different. What they have in common is that each provides for their country an overview of any major changes in policy during the twentieth century; and examines how practice on the ground impacted on the lives and experiences of people with intellectual disabilities, their families and others associated with them. And to bring this aspect to life, we asked authors to use one or more life stories. People interpreted this differently. Some authors chose to use a case study to provide the central narrative – see for example Danae Karydaki's chapter on Greece, with its focus on the notorious Island of Leros, and Guðrún Stefánsdóttir's on Iceland, built around the life story of her friend Ebba. Others have used life stories as short vignettes, illustrating different aspects of policy.

How we selected the countries

The selection of countries was in part deliberative, and in part serendipitous. A chapter on the UK, the home of both the editors, was a must, particularly as the absence of an authoritative history was the spark for the book in the first place. We agreed that a chapter on the USA was essential, given its influence over both eugenics and normalisation, the leading ideologies over the century. Its lead, as several chapters show, was followed by other Western countries, some might even say slavishly. We were delighted when Philip Ferguson agreed to emerge from retirement to write the USA chapter. So, the book includes the usual suspects, but we have also managed to roam far beyond them, by finding authors in Taiwan and Hong Kong, Ghana and Greece, the Czech Republic and Hungary. As we discuss below, intellectual disability history is a relatively young branch of the discipline, dating back to the 1980s even in the West, so we are immensely grateful to those authors who responded creatively and enthusiastically to our call. For some, it entailed a good deal of original scholarship, given the absence of any kind of historical narrative. The most striking instance is Ghana, where, as Auberon Jaleel Odoom and Jane Abraham's chapter indicates, intellectual disability was such a private matter until the late twentieth century that the condition barely had a name, and records are scanty. But even in Greece, where the Leros scandal took place, there has been no authoritative history – until now.

We have a sparkling set of chapters. Yes, they differ in the amount of detail, the extent to which they cover the whole twentieth century, the sophistication of the life stories, and the inclusion of narratives from people with more profound impairments, but they also provide unique transnational perspectives on a much neglected area of scholarship.

We are only too aware that this book leaves out so much. Canada, with its pioneering of retribution for eugenic excesses, and advocacy for individual budgets and brokerage. Ireland, where the history is entwined with a Catholic Church establishment whose reputation for care services is severely tarnished. The huge populations of India and China. The Spanish-speaking parts of the world. Norway, Sweden, Denmark and Finland, pioneers of normalisation, deinstitutionalisation and community living.... None of these are adequately represented.

What we have brought together here is but a start. Our hope is that what we have brought together here is the beginning of a more global perspective on the history of intellectual disability. Our intention has been to begin to view this history through a much wider lens than has been the case until now. May it inspire others to emulate what the contributors to this book have done.

The historiography of intellectual disability

The history of intellectual disability is a growing field of historical interest and yet the historiography remains limited. The most significant scholarly work is from the USA – James W. Trent produced a ground-breaking history of the nineteenth and twentieth centuries in the USA (Trent, 1994), while Ferguson contributed a rare historical account of people with profound and complex impairments (Ferguson, 1994). An important edited collection, Noll and Trent's *Mental Retardation in America: A reader* (New York, 2004) followed. Digby and Wright's *From Idiocy to Mental Deficiency* (1996) was the first significant historical work from the UK. Its focus is on the pre-asylum period from the Middle Ages to the nineteenth century. Bartlett and Wright's (1999) *Outside the Walls of the Asylum* was a history of care beyond institutions. And there has been a scholarly history of Western Australia (Cocks et al, 1996). Mark Jackson's *The Borderland of Imbecility* (2000) captures the intellectual underpinnings of the concept of feeble-mindedness at the turn of the century, while Matthew Thompson's (1998) *The Problem of Mental Deficiency* remains the definitive, and exceptional, account of the British Mental Deficiency Act of 1913, its causes and consequences.

McDonagh, Goodey and Stainton have published on pre-twentieth-century history from the Middle Ages, most recently with *Intellectual Disability: A conceptual history, 1200–1900* (2018), and specialists have emerged such as Irina Mezler on the medieval period (2018). There is work on eugenics and the asylum era in the USA, Canada, the UK and Nazi Germany but little related to modern policy and practice. The latest attempt at a global perspective is Michael L. Wehmeyer's collection *The Story of Intellectual Disability* (2013), heavily American dominated and with little about the influence of history on modern practice.

Hence there are significant gaps in the historical record, particularly perspectives from beyond the Anglosphere. Ironically, more progress has been made in the field of life stories, discussed below.

Life stories

The inclusion of life stories is a distinctive feature. Tales of policy can be quite dry, while how policy impacts, or does not impact, on individuals makes for a more interesting and too often untold story.

After all, what is the point of policy if not to impact on how people live, for better or worse?

Life stories began to feature in the way intellectual disability is known about over half a century ago. In England, Joey Deacon, resident of a long-stay hospital, published his life story in 1974, with the help of four friends. It created quite a stir. Joey appeared on children's TV, but also gave his name to a term of insult – 'Joey' – in use in playgrounds in England and Wales until the end of the twentieth century if not beyond.[1] American social scientists also pioneered life stories. Robert Edgerton's account of the lives of former residents of a large California institution drew on self-reported life stories (Edgerton, 1967), and Robert Bogdan and Steven Taylor published two important life stories in a book entitled 'Inside Out' (1982). Their conclusion was that the concept of 'mental retardation' was not only not useful; it was 'seriously misleading' (Bogdan and Taylor, 1982, reprinted 1989, p 76).

Life stories have flourished in the UK, including some serious oral history projects documenting life in institutions (Potts and Fido, 1991; Keilty and Woodley, 2013). Interest was sustained through the work of the Open University's Social History of Learning Disability Group of which both editors are members. The group has published individual life stories, including of celebrated campaigner Mabel Cooper (Cooper, 1997), and accounts by families of their experiences in different policy eras (Rolph et al, 2005). Mabel Cooper's story influenced wider agendas, including inspiring young people in schools (Walmsley et al, 2017), an exhibition in a London museum, and a widely acclaimed immersive theatre production performed in London in 2018 (Ledger and Walmsley, forthcoming). Attention has been paid to the mechanics and ethics of life-story writing, with discussion over who has ownership and how far life stories can be 'used' by academics to make a point rather than stand as testimony in their own right (Walmsley, 1995; Booth and Booth, 1998; Atkinson and Walmsley, 1999, 2010). Some of this intense interest has percolated to other countries, often influenced by personal relationships between the academics concerned. Life stories have been recorded from Australia (Manning, 2010), Iceland (Stefansdóttir and Traustadóttir, 2015), Ireland (Hamilton and Atkinson, 2009; Kearney with Johnson, 2009) and Austria (Koenig, 2012), and there have been some significant anthologies (Atkinson et al, 2000; Traustadóttir and Johnson, 2000; Johnson and Traustadóttir, 2005), the latter two international in scope.

The life stories in this collection vary widely, both in how they were collected and how they are used. As editors, we did not stipulate how the stories were to be found, or how much say the person whose story is told has over its use. This, we reckoned, would be a step too far in countries where there has been no tradition of recording the stories of people with intellectual disabilities or their families. Not to mention the strict word limits people were working to. We did emphasise the importance of actually hearing, rather than hearing about, people's voices and experiences. The result has been immensely pleasing: the stories throughout the book are both respectful and powerful. Authors have taken differing stances, some using the stories to build the chapter (Australia, Iceland, Taiwan, the USA), others using them as an illustrative vignette (Ghana, Greece, Hungary), while others have done a mixture (the UK). Some use stories to illustrate change over time (Australia, Iceland, the UK, the USA), drawing on existing scholarship, but that has not been possible where there has been no recording of life stories until now, hence others use the stories to illustrate contrasting fortunes of people alive now (Czech Republic, Hong Kong, Hungary, Taiwan). It is particularly gratifying that work on the book inspired some authors to begin life history research. We very much hope that this will be a sustained benefit of the transnational cooperation initiated by working on the book.

Of course, under the constraints of an edited volume with strict word limits, much has not been achieved. Family advocacy was the start of change in many of the countries whose history is described, and it would have been ideal to include more family members' accounts, along the lines pioneered by Rolph et al (2005). Similarly, most of the life stories are of people who would probably be regarded as having mild or moderate intellectual disabilities. As so often, the voices of people with more profound intellectual disabilities are too quiet, or absent altogether. However, we are pleased to have made a start and hope our work sets a direction that others can build on.

Language

The language of intellectual disability is, as one group of historians described it, 'remarkably unstable', the instability arising from there being 'no definitive trans-historical concept of intellectual disability' (McDonagh et al, 2018, 2). Those we define as intellectually disabled today cannot be traced back in a straight line to an identical group labelled as 'idiots' in the eighteenth century, even less so to the 'idiotic' of the Middle Ages, which essentially described the lower orders of society as a whole. Language to describe the group deemed to lack intellectual faculty has passed with extraordinary speed through 'idiot', 'moron', 'mentally deficient', 'cretin', 'mental defective', 'sub-normal', 'mentally handicapped', 'learning disabled', 'learning difficulty', 'cognitive disability', 'developmental disability' and many more. 'Intellectual disability' is just the most recent. This is more than just the natural evolution of language over time, and more than the necessary replacement of words such as 'moron' and 'cretin' which have made the short journey from medical category to street insult. Firstly, those we define as belonging to this group over time change, due to cultural and social ideas about what constitutes lack of mental faculty; how important this is considered to be at any given time; how much of a factor 'intelligence' is deemed to be in belonging to society; and whether lack of intellect is considered a threat or viewed without alarm. Secondly, who are defined as intellectually disabled is the subject of power claims, expressed through language, by the professional groups that seek the authority to understand, own and control them. Each change of label is a professional claim to authority, by doctors, social workers, psychologists, advocates, policy makers, historians or whoever else wishes to stake their claim.

The matter of language becomes even more complex, and interesting, in a transnational study such as this one. The debate so far has been about the contortions through which the English language has travelled, and continues to travel. In the Anglosphere in modern times we have insisted on a construction such as 'people with an intellectual disability' to make the point that someone is a person first and has a disability second. We find that in Mandarin Chinese and Hungarian the construction 'people with a ...' can simply not be formed. In Mandarin the construction has to be 'intellectually (or mentally) disabled person', while in Hungarian a tortuous construction that translates as 'person living with a mental disability' has to be used. In Greece a term which translates literally as 'small-minded' ('μικρονοϊκός' – usually translated as 'feeble-minded') was used up to the 1980s by practitioners. Within major Ghanaian languages there are specific negative words, for example 'Asotowo' (meaning 'idiot' in Ewe) and 'Buulu' (meaning 'stupid' in Ga), while those with Down's Syndrome are labelled 'nsuoba' meaning spirit or water children in Twi. As Hungarian contributor Ágnes Turnpenny commented, 'what is interesting is the struggle for defining the "right" terminology and which group gets to control the language of disability. Very often this is a symbolic act in itself: attempts to adapt and enforce terms perceived as "progressive" usually translated from foreign languages – German or English.' This obsession with language, she argues, distracts from the focus on real exclusionary policy and practice – institutions, guardianship, poverty and so on.

Eugenics

No history of intellectual disability in the twentieth century can be written without acknowledgement of the influence of the 'science' of eugenics (meaning 'well born' in Greek). First framed by Darwin's half-cousin Francis Galton in 1863, it advocated that degeneration of the racial stock in advanced countries was caused by hereditary defect resulting from uncontrolled breeding by the poorer classes. Idiocy, along with mental ill-health, criminality, alcoholism, physical frailty and prostitution, all resulted from uncontrolled and irresponsible breeding – idiocy became synonymous with criminality and promiscuity. The situation could only be addressed by encouraging breeding among the wealthier, healthier classes (positive eugenics) or reducing breeding by the 'degenerate' classes, through segregation, birth control, sterilisation or even euthanasia (negative eugenics). By the early twentieth century eugenics movements were strong in the Anglosphere and much of Europe, particularly the Nordic countries, and exerted a strong influence on both policy and practice.

However, this collection shows that eugenic science cannot be used as a catch-all explanation of early-twentieth-century policy and practice towards people with intellectual disabilities. Other forces were at work, both outside and inside the Anglosphere and Europe. In Taiwan and Ghana, for example, traditional belief systems entwined with economic anxieties to engender similar hostilities, independent of Social Darwinist catastrophising. In communist Hungary and Czechoslovakia it was the fetishisation of proletarian labour that created a dividing line of belonging between the moderately disabled, who could work, and the severely disabled, who could not. In Europe and the English-speaking world anxieties about the challenges of modernity and what constituted a modern citizen gave rise to a distrust of, and even fear for the well-being of, the citizen who seemed to lack capacity. In Greece patriotic social movements fed off anxieties about the breakdown of traditional community and hierarchies just as much as they embraced the ideology of degeneration. Eugenics has its place in the history of intellectual disability, but it does not own it.

Overview of chapters

In any collection of this nature there is much debate about the ordering and grouping of chapters. There was a temptation to group contributions in a conventional geopolitical way – the Anglosphere, Western Europe, Eastern Europe, the East, Africa. We decided consciously not to follow that temptation. For us as editors, part of the fascination of the book is the surprising connections and divergences that our contributors describe across space, time and culture. For this reason, we have ordered chapters alphabetically by name of country, and allowed both the links and disconnections to speak for themselves. This has had the unintended but, for us, happy consequence of leaving the United Kingdom and the United States, usually foregrounded in studies of intellectual disability, as the final chapters: a placement which immediately subverts and challenges our mental ordering of ideas about intellectual disability in the twentieth-century world.

The chapters

Lee-Ann Monk's narrative of intellectual disability in **Australia** is viewed through the lens of Kew Cottages, one of the country's most significant institutions, built in 1887, modelled on English 'idiot' asylums, and which did not close until 2008. As part of the Anglosphere, the development of policy and practice over this time in Australia was deeply intertwined with the UK and the USA; a eugenic discourse, post-war stagnation and then a tortuous journey to deinstitutionalisation. The nexus between policy and practice, and the sheer power of the institution is brilliantly captured through the life stories of two individuals, one of whom (literally) battled his way from Kew back into the community, not least by joining the Australian armed forces in the Second World War, the other who passed decades in the institution despite national publicity about his fate and the drive for normalisation.

Across any history of **Austria** in this period will fall the long and murderous shadow of the mass-elimination programme of 'unworthy life' that took place after the Nazi *anschluss* (connection), or annexation, in 1938. Yet as Gertraud Kremsner, Oliver Koenig and Tobias Buchner demonstrate starkly, these killing programmes 'did not appear from nowhere'. Reformism after the First World War had been buried under the strains of massive economic recession and a radical strain of eugenic thought that framed the 'unfit' and the 'inferior' as worthy targets of euthanasia and sterilisation. The ingredients were already in place for a disastrous genocidal collaboration between the medical establishment and Nazi officialdom. Failure to reform at the end of the war led to the continuation of institutional models and even the return of some National Socialist perpetrators to their positions in the Austrian medical establishment. Only in 1986 did a serious deinstitutionalisation programme begin for people with intellectual disabilities, and a system of economisation and managerialism remains a barrier to independence and liberation today.

The global upheavals of the twentieth century are deeply imprinted on the land we know today as the **Czech Republic**. It was first part of the Austro-Hungarian Empire, then from 1918 became the republic of Czechoslavakia, suffered Nazi occupation from 1938 to 1945, emerged a communist state from 1948, and then, after its 'Velvet Revolution' and a split from Slovakia, became the democratic, Western-oriented Czech Republic. Monika Mužáková and Iva Strnadová's account of the lives of people with intellectual disabilities through the prism of these events ably demonstrates that marginalisation does not leave people isolated from and immune to political upheavals, but rather often places them at the centre. They describe a battle between eugenicists and a group of liberal educators in the inter-war period (largely won by the educators, who at least curbed eugenic excesses), the horror of targeted extermination under Nazism, and a communist regime that rewarded those with mild or moderate disabilities who could work, and discriminated against and marginalised the severely disabled. Changes in social care provision and education policy post-Velvet Revolution offer hope of greater inclusion and support in the future.

Jane Abraham and Auberon Jaleel Odoom recount, for the first time, the twentieth-century history of intellectual disability in **Ghana**. the first sub-Saharan British colony to achieve independence (in 1957). The story is of a stark clash between the beliefs of modernity and the long-standing beliefs of a society on which modernity seeks to impose itself. In traditional, rural Ghanaian society, the mildly or moderately intellectually disabled person could integrate with relative ease into a labour-intensive agricultural economy, where literacy was not at a premium. For the severely or profoundly disabled person, life was less predictable. Seclusion or even infanticide arose from spiritual beliefs about the influence of evil forces or punishment from the gods. Beneath these beliefs lay economic concerns about families bearing the load of an unproductive person, allocating precious financial resources to the education of a person seen as unlikely to benefit from it, and anxieties about marriageability. Two illuminating life stories suggest that people with intellectual disabilities in Ghana are learning to manage and resist these cultural complexities and assert their own identities.

In her groundbreaking account of **Greece**, Danae Karydaki gives the first historical account (including first-hand life stories) of the scandal of the Leros island asylums, which erupted in a British press exposé in 1989. Karydaki frames the story of intellectual disability in Greece in the twentieth century around this 'island of outcasts'. The origins of Leros as a dumping ground for the 'idiot' detritus of the mainland can be traced to the Greek civil war, urbanisation trends pressurising traditional social structures, and patriotic social movements between the two world wars. Karydaki paints a vision of society's magnetic attraction to the island as the ultimate site of incarceration for those who are unwanted, and reminds us that for those inside, the prison and the asylum are indistinguishable. She draws out the process of infantilisation of the adult person that must take place for us to consign people to the unchanging Neverland of the total institution.

Another site of twentieth-century upheaval (was anywhere not turbulent?) was **Hong Kong**, the world's most densely populated area, a British colony until 1997, when it became a special administrative region of the People's Republic of China. Phyllis King Shui Wong traces the journey from the earliest service provision of the 1970s, through a 'golden period' in the 1990s when it seemed that a new age of rights and family- and self-advocacy was dawning, to a worrying period of minimal progress and stagnation that threatens to submerge earlier gains. The moving life stories she gathered track this trajectory from defiance and struggle in the early days, through the euphoria of progress and change, to the present state of anxiety as victory appears in danger of receding.

Like the Czech Republic, **Hungary** endured a century of extreme turbulence, in which it veered from subject-part of empire to independence, Nazi occupation, communist dictatorship, and post-Communist democratisation. Ágnes Turnpenny skillfully draws out the impact of these political upheavals on the population labelled as intellectually disabled. The population faced 'extreme and shocking' poverty in the early part of the century with licensed begging for those without family or institution, a highly racialised form of eugenics in the inter-war period, and extermination and starvation under Nazi occupation. Under the post-war communist regime, the 'workshy' severely disabled population was marginalised into institutions, and state support withdrawn from families who persisted in the care of the 'hindrance' that was their 'ineducable' disabled child. Post-communist hope of a better future, particularly after EU accession and the adoption of human rights policies, now seems premature as institutions stubbornly persist. A fascinating sub-text is the desperation of Hungarian policy makers to align themselves with the West, 'catching up forever', and distancing themselves from neighbouring countries with which they do not wish to be associated.

An intriguing story emerges from **Iceland**, a country with a population of less than 350,000. Guðrún Stefánsdóttir draws out the ambivalent legacy of normalisation, a theory for integration emanating in the main from Denmark and Sweden, and heavily influential in the Nordic world including Iceland. Does this approach offer a gateway to inclusion, or does it put pressure on individuals to learn adaptive behaviour to achieve conditional acceptance, while oppressive behaviour remains unchallenged? Why, despite the adoption of normalisation, did segregation remain common in Nordic countries? The life story of Eygló (Ebba) Hreinsdóttir illustrates the conflicting effects normalisation principles could have on the life of an intellectually disabled person. Thanks to these normalisation ideas Ebba escaped the institution, only to find herself in a new conflict to resist pressure to become a 'normal' woman, and to assert herself as an individual – a battle which, eventually, she won. Her story also brings out in human terms the painful legacy of the eugenic policy of involuntary sterilisation, enacted into Icelandic law in 1938, and the practice of which persisted into the 1980s.

Back in the Anglosphere, **New Zealand** entered the twentieth century with a burgeoning asylum system, an 1899 Immigration Act prohibiting 'idiot persons', a growing eugenics movement and a lust for the confinement of the difficult and the different. New Zealand's Mental Defectives Act of 1911 preceded the British Mental Deficiency Act by two years. Carol Hamilton demonstrates how even from the gloomiest depths of institutionalisation, neglect and indifference, positive reform of policy and practice, and great improvements in people's lived experience, can occur. An anti-institutionalisation movement began early in post-war New Zealand and by the end of the century there had been a paradigm shift in ideas about how and where people labelled intellectually disabled should live. While problems and challenges remain, and the reform movement goes on, the success of the deinstitutionalisation movement that Hamilton describes should not be underestimated.

Taiwan emerged from Japanese colonisation in 1945, was then governed by the Republic of China, and after the 1948 communist revolution in China became the seat of government of the ousted Republic of China government. Yueh-Ching Chou recounts a fascinating story, through the life stories of those who lived through the times, of small amounts of institutional care from the 1950s, the beginnings of community service provision in the 1980s, the persistence of sterilisation 'solutions', the emergence of a powerful self-advocacy movement and a society in which 90% of people with intellectual disabilities still live in the family home. Fewer than 0.5% live independently in the community. The status of people with intellectual disabilities is complicated by social factors such as the mass migration of over one million people from China after the civil war, of whom 600,000 were army veterans. Their low social status entwined the fates of these exiles and people with disabilities. This complex story illustrates how a marginalising discourse can emerge without influence from the eugenic theories of the Anglosphere and Europe.

We end where we usually begin, with the **United Kingdom** and the **United States**. It is salutary to see these countries as part of a global story which is interconnected but also disparate, with influences other than their own at work. We argue that in the first half of the twentieth century UK policy was not driven solely by eugenic discourse but by a commonly held assumption across the ideological spectrum that the 'mentally deficient' population needed 'fixing' in some way. Lurking beneath this desire for completeness and the tidying-up of the social sphere were deep anxieties about urban modernity and human capacity to meet its challenges. In the second half of the century we see the voice of the person with intellectual disability finally emerge, as the institutions met their end. As in Hong Kong there was a 'golden period' in the 1990s when thoughtful policy allowed hopes of inclusion and a better tomorrow to soar. The authors end with a cautionary warning from the twenty-first century, where gains seem to be receding and the institution rising from its grave. Philip Ferguson's masterly succinct summary of the American century uses the stories of three families, the 'Kallikaks', the Kennedys and the Fergusons. The fictitious Kallikaks were used as part of the vicious eugenic libel against the intellectually disabled population that stoked the cruel mass institutionalisation programmes of the early century. Ferguson tells the story of Emma Wolverton, one of those on whose life stories the mythical Kallikaks were based and created to spread fear and drive segregational policy. The story of the famous Kennedys shows the post-war journey of the intellectually disabled person from a hidden site of shame to the policy reforms of the community return. Finally, the story of Philip's own Ferguson family shows some of the great post-reform liberating shifts towards a life of choice and inclusion that have taken place, and alerts us to the brooding threats that still lurk.

Transnational themes

One of the benefits of a collection such as this is that it offers fresh insights. Here we seek to highlight these, while recognising that readers may make connections we have not spotted.

Families

A feature common to all countries represented here is the importance of families. Until the later twentieth century, intellectual disability was a private matter, for families and local communities in Ghana, Taiwan and Hong Kong. Even in Europe our authors point out that in Greece and Hungary it was seen as a family responsibility until well into the twentieth century. In those countries influenced by the United States – the UK, Australia, New Zealand – despite the rhetoric, families remained the mainstay of support throughout the institutional era. And those souls who ended up in Leros (Greece) were the ones who had no family to support or defend them. Despite the appearance of official interest in people with intellectual disability, particularly children, in all the countries represented here, families remain the most significant source of support.

It is also striking that across the world represented in this book it was families who were at the forefront of agitating for reform, for alternatives to institutions, for educational opportunities and for changing attitudes to their relatives. It takes courage to stand up and fight for your child, especially in societies where those children are stigmatised – and that is the case in all the societies represented here. Particularly striking was the resistance to the murder taking place in Austria under the Nazis, but also the courage of the families who challenged authorities in Czechoslovakia, Hong Kong and Taiwan, and the determination of some families in Hungary to care for their children despite incurring the wrath of the state for doing so.

Our book also reminds us that at times families are less than benign. Some resist deinstitutionalisation. Some set up and defend services which themselves become outdated. In extreme cases, they allow people with more severe impairments to die.

Exclusion and inequality

This collection shows us how globally, across geographical borders, cultures, language, ideologies and class, those labelled as intellectually disabled are a presence, and they matter both as subject and object, influencer and receiver of policy and practice. They are almost always, but not inevitably, an out-group against whom in-groups define themselves. Policy, as in the first half of the century, sometimes embraces this exclusion, culminating in the despicable savagery of Nazi killing programmes, but with many other manifestations: the asylum; involuntary sterilisation; the persecution of those unfit to work; special schooling that is the first irrevocable step in a lifetime on the outside without hope. In the latter half of the century, policy has bent towards the soft words of inclusion, integration, non-discrimination, rights and opportunity.

In every country whose history is described, people with intellectual disabilities are an out-group, looked down upon and excluded. Goodey (2011) ascribes this to the fetishisation of intelligence in modern societies. However, particularly in Ghana for example, it seems to be as much a product of inability to make an economic contribution, and this was also the case for more severely impaired individuals in the Eastern bloc countries, Czechoslovakia and Hungary, under Communist governments (late 1940s to 1989). The boundaries of the out-group have varied, influenced by social, economic and political conditions. In societies where subsistence agriculture is dominant, people with mild or moderate impairments can indeed get by, contribute and be part of society. This was also true in Communist Hungary and Czechoslovakia, where full employment of those able to work was a state priority. And in other countries during wartime when labour was needed, as Gelb (2004) showed in relation to the USA. But, depressingly, in no country whose history is narrated here have people with more severe impairments been included as equal citizens.

The march of progress?

How far does this book uphold what was a widespread view in the lifetime of both editors, that things are getting better for people with intellectual disabilities? It is a moot point whether leaving intellectual disability as a private and hidden issue is preferable to being identified and 'treated'. Educational opportunities are welcome, but coming to the attention of officialdom in Austria after 1938 was a potential death sentence, and even in those places where euthanasia was not practised, being labelled could mean many years of incarceration.

Lee-Ann Monk points to the paradox that freedom was achieved in the early twentieth century more readily than in the later deinstitutionalisation era. While there are some optimistic pointers including the closure of large-scale institutions in the Anglosphere and Scandinavia and the development of self-advocacy in Taiwan and Hong Kong, several authors identify the late twentieth century as a high point, with a falling away since (Hong Kong and the UK), and where they have existed, institutions prove themselves to be remarkably persistent. Furthermore, there is a marked legacy of eugenic ideas in relation to the fertility of women, even after the overt practice of sterilisation ends. Abortion of disabled foetuses is routine in some countries. As the life stories show, the strength of the nexus between policy and practice can often be cruelly disappointing. Even as gains are made, threats to reverse them slowly take shape on the horizon.

Human rights and the UN Convention on the Rights of Persons with Disabilities

One of the arguments for this book was that most (not quite all) countries represented here are signatories of the UN Convention on the Rights of Persons with Disabilities (UNCRPD). The Convention makes a number of statements which indicate that all are committed to rights-based policy and practice. One of the paradoxes, however, is that such statements fly in the face of the very different histories represented in this book, and across the world. The fact that the UK, one of the countries that has taken deinstitutionalisation and independent living furthest (McDonagh et al, 2018), has been taken to task for failing to uphold it (UN Committee on the Rights of Persons with Disabilities, 2016) perhaps illustrates what an ambitious task it is to get countries across the world, with very contrasting histories and cultural influences, to bring policy and practice in line with the Convention. Without going into further depth, our contribution is to suggest that without understanding the history of intellectual disabilities in different countries it is unrealistic to enact a Convention which reflects Western ideas of what is best for disabled people.

What next?

As editors, we are only too aware that this book is just the start of a movement to understand intellectual disability in a transnational and historical context. So many countries are not included. Many voices remain unheard, particularly the voices of those whose impairments are more severe. We intend to do more ourselves, and hope that our example will inspire others to follow our lead, to record the twentieth-century history of intellectual disabilities in countries across the world.

The book perhaps raises more questions than answers, about both the countries it features and those it does not feature. Questions about resistance to the dehumanising of people with intellectual disabilities, about what prompts and sustains it. Questions about what justifies exclusion and control where the language of eugenics is not spoken. Questions about the role of technology and medical advances, the implications of prenatal testing and abortion, the potential of personalisation and individual budgets to break the depressing cycle of low investment, scandal, reform and progressive promise. If the book gives rise to such questions in the minds of the editors, we hope that it will spark more reflection in our readers.

In compiling this book, we have consciously ignored 'Nothing about us without us', the slogan of the disabled people's movement in the UK. This book is *about* people with intellectual disabilities, not *by* them, and we have not as yet attempted to make it more accessible; it is important that we do so by sharing its key messages in a way that at least some people with intellectual disabilities can understand.

The last word in this Introduction is inspired by Ted Rowe, one of the men whose story is told. Part of his escape from the institution involved putting his life on the line in the Second World War. We must all be prepared to put ourselves on the line to shape societies in which all humans can take their place without question, without conditions, and without labels that put a ceiling over them from the moment of birth.

Acknowledgement

The editors would like to thank the anonymous referee of the manuscript for his or her insightful suggestions, many of which have been incorporated here.

Note

[1] This webpage gives a good summary of Joey's significance: www.tpas. cymru/blog/joey-deacons-life-his-birthday-and-his-impact-on-me

References

Atkinson, D. and Walmsley, J. (1999) 'Using auto/biographical approaches with people with learning difficulties', *Disability & Society*, 14(2), 203–16.

Atkinson, D. and Walmsley, J. (2010) 'History from the inside: Towards an inclusive history of learning disability', *Scandinavian Journal of Disability Research*, 12(4), 273–86.

Atkinson, D., McCarthy, M. et al (2000) *Good times, bad times: Women with learning difficulties tell their stories*, Kidderminster: BILD Publications.

Bartlett, P. and Wright, D. (1999) *Outside the walls of the asylum: The history of care in the community 1750–2000*, London, Athlone Press.

Bogdan, R. and Taylor, S. (1982) *Inside out: The social meaning of retardation*, Toronto: University of Toronto Press.

Booth, T. and Booth, W. (1998) *Growing up with parents who have learning disabilities*, London: Routledge.

Cocks, E., Fox, C., Brogan, M. and Lee, M. (eds) (1996) *Under blue skies: The social construction of intellectual disability in Western Australia*, Perth, WA: Edith Cowan University.

Cooper, M. (1997) 'Mabel Cooper's life story' in D. Atkinson, M. Jackson and J. Walmsley (eds) *Forgotten lives: Exploring the history of learning disability*, Kidderminster: BILD.

Deacon, J. (1974) *Tongue tied: Fifty years of friendship in a subnormality hospital*, London, National Society for Mentally Handicapped Children.

Digby, A. and Wright, D. (eds) (1996) *From idiocy to mental deficiency: Historical perspectives on people with learning disabilities*, London, Routledge.

Edgerton, R. (1967) *The cloak of competence: Stigma in the lives of the mentally retarded*, Berkeley, University of California Press.

Ferguson, P.M. (1994) *Abandoned to their fate: Social policy and practice towards severely retarded people in America 1820–1920*, Philadelphia, Temple University Press.

Gelb, S.A. (2004) '"Mental deficients" fighting fascism: the unplanned normalization of World War II' in S. Noll and J.W. Trent Jr (eds), *Mental retardation in America: A historical reader*, New York, New York University Press, 308–21.

Goodey, C.F. (2011) *A history of intelligence and 'intellectual disability': The shaping of psychology in early modern Europe*, Farnham: Ashgate.

Hamilton, C. and Atkinson, D. (2009) '"A Story to Tell": learning from the life-stories of older people with intellectual disabilities in Ireland', *British Journal of Learning Disabilities*, 37(4), 316–22.

Jackson, M. (2000) *The borderland of imbecility: Medicine, society and the fabrication of the feeble mind in late-Victorian and Edwardian England*, Manchester: Manchester University Press.

Johnson, K. and Traustadottir, R. (eds) (2005) *Deinstitutionalisation and people with intellectual disabilities: In and out of institutions*, London: Jessica Kingsley.

Kearney, P. with Johnson, K. (2009) *This was my life, I'm here to tell it: The life and times of Patrick Kearney*, Ennis, Co. Clare: Brothers of Charity Inclusive Research Group.

Keilty, T. and Woodley, K. (2013) *No going back*, Sheffield: Centre for Welfare Reform.

Koenig, O. (2012) 'Any added value? Co-constructing life stories of and with people with intellectual disabilities', *British Journal of Learning Disabilities*, 40(3), 213–21.

Ledger, S. and Walmsley, J. (forthcoming) '"The Madhouse": Working with performance artists with learning disabilities to share the history of institutions and increase public awareness and involvement in activism', in K. Johnson and K. Soldatic (eds) *Global perspectives on disability activism and advocacy*, Melbourne: Routledge.

Manning, C. (2010) '"My memory's back!" Inclusive learning disability research using ethics, oral history and digital storytelling', *British Journal of Learning Disabilities*, 38(3), 160–7.

McDonagh, P., Goodey, C.F. and Stainton, T. (eds) (2018) *Intellectual disability: A conceptual history, 1200–1900*, Manchester: Manchester University Press.

Mezler, I. (2018) *Fools and idiots? Intellectual disability in the Middle Ages*, Manchester: Manchester University Press.

Noll, S. and Trent, J.W. Jnr (eds) (2004) *Mental retardation in America: A historical reader*, New York, New York University Press.

Potts, M. and Fido, R. (1991) *A fit person to be removed: Personal accounts of life in a mental deficiency institution*, Northcote: Plymouth.

Rolph S., Atkinson, D., Nind, M. and Welshman, J. (2005) *Witnesses to change: Families, learning difficulties and history*, Kidderminster: BILD Publications.

Stefánsdóttir, G.V. and Traustadóttir, R. (2015) 'Life histories as counter-narratives against dominant and negative stereotypes about people with intellectual disabilities', *Disability & Society*, 30(3), 368–80.

Thompson, M. (1998) *The problem of mental deficiency: Eugenics, democracy and social policy in Britain, c. 1870–1959*, Oxford: Oxford University Press.

Traustadóttir, R. and Johnson, K. (eds) (2000) *Women with learning disabilities: Finding a place in the world*, London: Jessica Kingsley Press.

Trent, J.W. Jnr (1994) *Inventing the feeble mind: A history of mental retardation in the United States*, Berkeley: University of California Press.

UN Committee on the Rights of Persons with Disabilities (2016) *Inquiry concerning the United Kingdom of Great Britain and Northern Ireland carried out by the Committee under article 6 of the Optional Protocol to the Convention Report of the Committee*, New York: United Nations, available at: www.ohchr.org/EN/HRBodies/CRPD/Pages/InquiryProcedure.aspx [accessed 21/2/17].

Walmsley, J. (1995) 'Life history interviews with people with learning disabilities', *Oral History*, 23(1), 71–7.

Walmsley, J., Ledger, S., Christian, P. and Jayne, Z. (2017) 'How come we didn't know all this stuff happened: using mixed media to tell young people with learning disabilities the history of institutions', Presentation at Social History of Learning Disability Conference, Milton Keynes, July 2017.

Wehmeyer, M. (ed) (2013) *The story of intellectual disability*, Baltimore: Brookes.

Welshman, J. and Walmsley, J. (eds) (2006) *Care, control and citizenship*, London: Palgrave.

ONE

Paradoxical lives: intellectual disability policy and practice in twentieth-century Australia

Lee-Ann Monk

Introduction

In 1911, in a paper read at the Australasian Medical Congress, Melbourne doctor J.W.Y. Fishbourne urged Australia to implement policies to remedy 'the problem of the feeble-minded'. In failing to act, he asserted, the nation was lagging behind international opinion: 'The United States of America recognise the danger and England is beginning to waken up to the seriousness of the problem'. To prove his point, he cited evidence from recent British and American investigations and quoted the opinions of Dr Martin Barr, Chief Physician of the Pennsylvania School for Feeble-Minded, and Mary Dendy, English social reformer, both of whom advocated permanent segregation of those deemed feeble-minded (Fishbourne, 1913). As this example suggests, international ideas have influenced Australian thinking on intellectual disabilities. As a consequence, the broad outline of Australia's policy history follows a similar pattern to other Western countries. In the first half of the twentieth century, eugenic anxieties about the 'menace of the feeble-minded' dominated thinking, as they did across the Western world. Policy consequently emphasised institutional segregation. After the Second World War, new optimism about the developmental potential of people with intellectual disabilities saw the emphasis shift from institutional segregation to community integration. The shift was underpinned by the philosophy of normalisation, which dominated Australian policy from the 1970s. Combined with the desire of governments to reduce costs, it resulted in policies of deinstitutionalisation which saw institutions for people with intellectual disabilities begin to close from the early 1980s (see Earl, 2018).

In Australia, state governments were responsible for health and education services (Earl, 2018, 308). To explore the impact of policy on people in Australia, this chapter focuses on the experiences of people admitted to Kew Cottages, one of the most significant institutions for people with intellectual disabilities. Opened in 1887, the Cottages were the first major policy response of the government of Victoria to the care of children with intellectual disabilities. Modelled on English 'idiot' asylums, the establishment of the Kew Idiot Asylum, as the Cottages were first known, reflected the then prevailing optimism about the potential of people with intellectual disabilities (Monk and Manning, 2012). The first purpose-built institution for people with intellectual disabilities in Australia, the Cottages grew into one of the largest before closing in 2008. Thus, their history spans the twentieth century. The life stories of their residents offer a lens through which to explore how policy impacted people's lives. In addition to archival sources, the chapter draws on oral history interviews with Kew residents, conducted by Corinne Manning in 2005 and 2006 as part of a research project exploring the history of the Cottages (Manning, 2008; 2010).

'The problem of the feeble-minded'

Five-year-old Ted Rowe arrived at the Children's Cottages in March 1925. Found abandoned on the streets of Melbourne as an infant, he had spent the years since in the care of the Children's Welfare Department. But in early 1925, the staff at that Department's Children's Depot concluded that theirs was no longer the appropriate institution for him. In certificates seeking his admission to the Cottages, the Matron declared that he was 'idiotic in his behaviour, irritable and inclined to hurt other children and cannot be taught habits of cleanliness and intelligence'. In her opinion, he showed 'no capacity for being taught anything'. The two doctors called to examine him, as the law required, agreed: both thought his physical appearance and behaviour were indicative of 'idiocy'. His behaviour they deemed inappropriate for his age, noting his apparent inability to speak more than 'a few words' and his tendency to laugh 'merrily at everything and nothing'. And so, on a sunny autumn day in March, Ted made the journey from the Children's Depot across the Yarra River to the Children's Cottages, where he would remain for the next eight years (PROV, VPRS 7565/P1, Unit 7).

His progress quickly proved the Matron's assessment wrong. Within weeks he had learned the habits of cleanliness she had asserted he could not be taught, and could understand 'simple directions'. Ten months later he was, according to his case history: 'Considerably improved. Clean in habits.' Accompanying photographs seemingly attest that he was a 'Happy little chap'. By 1932, he was 'Getting on well' at the school (Department of Human Services, Victoria Archives, A/S 92/184/4). However, as Fishbourne's 1911 remarks suggest, by the time of Ted's admission, the optimism that had seen the Idiot Asylum established had dissipated, replaced by the conviction that the feeble-minded were, by virtue of hereditary 'defect', the cause of a multitude of social problems (Monk and Manning, 2012). While this belief found considerable support in Australia (Jones, 1999), it was slow to translate into policy in Victoria, despite widespread agreement about the need for action. In 1913 the government had established a day school for feeble-minded children in the suburb of Fitzroy, followed in 1915 by a second in another suburb, Montague. It had not, however, moved to enact legislation nor establish the residential institutions advocates considered necessary (Lewis, 1989). Consequently, when Ted arrived at the Children's Cottages, it was the only such residential institution in Victoria. In 1925, it was home to 378 residents (Report of the Inspector General of the Insane 1925, 4).

His admission coincided with a renewed push by government to counter the 'menace of the feeble-minded'. In 1926, the government introduced a Mental Deficiency Bill into parliament. Drawing considerably from the British Mental Deficiency Act 1913 as well as legislation recently enacted in Tasmania, the Bill set out 'a comprehensive scheme for the control, care and training of mental defectives of all classes' (Argyle, 1926; Jones, 1999, 319-42). To provide for the institutional segregation the Lunacy Department, the government department responsible for mental deficiency, purchased 'Travancore', a property in the Melbourne suburb of Flemington (Lewis, 1989, 269–70), with the intention of establishing:

> a residential school for quite young children, who might be described as high-grade mentally [sic] defectives … It was intended that children not younger than six years nor over the age of twelve years should be admitted, and that if they were considered suitable they would be retained there until, approximately, sixteen years of age. (Report of the Inspector-General of the Insane 1926, 39)

The school was intended to be one element in the system of control for, as the head of the Lunacy Department explained, on reaching the age of 16, pupils would be 'so classified that their future could be arranged for by boarding out or being sent on to the next type of institution, which it is intended should partake of the nature of a residential colony'. For this purpose, the Department had acquired a second property, 'ideally placed for the purposes of a farming and industrial colony for adult defectives'. The Cottages were to be reserved 'for the lower grade of mental defective, that is to say the idiot and imbecile of low type' (Report of the Inspector-General of the Insane 1926, 39). While the pressure of other business saw the Bill which precipitated its purchase lapse (Argyle, 1929, 800), Travancore Special School, duly renovated and equipped, opened in February 1933 (Report of the Inspector-General of the Insane 1933, 24). A month later, Ted was transferred there on 'trial leave' from the Cottages.

The record of his time at Travancore is sparse, recording only his IQ and that he was a 'Nice lad. Improving' (PROV, VPRS 7491/ P1). Ted, however, declared that he "liked Travancore it was a lovely place ... All the people were nice there". He recalled an "Open Day when parents visited to see what their children were doing and the children put on a show for them in the hall" (Rowe, 2006). Press reporting of similar occasions reflects keen public interest in the work of the school. In 1934, it welcomed a visit by the Victorian Women Citizens' Movement, who observed the children 'engaged in pastel work and other handcrafts, in reading and geography lessons' before being entertained by a 'short concert' (Age, 27 June 1934). Two years later, the Age marvelled at the 'high standard' of work at an exhibition of the children's handcrafts. 'Of special interest, too, was the vegetable stall, where produce grown by the senior boys', among whom Ted must have numbered, was for sale (Age, 20 November 1936, 24).

In 1937 Ted, now aged 16, was transferred once more, to the country town of Stawell where the government had opened a second residential institution, the Pleasant Creek Special School. By 1941, he was one of 'twelve boys' from the school 'in employment' (Report of the Director of Mental Hygiene 1941; NAA: B884, V240186; Rowe, 2006). Ted had been keen to work but "hated" the job the Department found him as a farm labourer. The farmer drove him "mad, he was a slave driver.... He wouldn't let you rest, when I sat down for a while he'd say, 'come on get up it's time to go to work'. They used to have a one-horse plough and I used to plough, sometimes at night-time till about midnight and on my own" (Rowe, 2006). While other young men returned to the institution, Ted lived on the property during the week, sleeping in a hut, away from the farmhouse. "I ended up buying a bike and I used to push myself into the store on it. I'd go into the store and see people in there on the weekend" (Report of the Director of Mental Hygiene 1941, 16; Rowe, 2006).

Ted, and other employed inmates faced a particular dilemma in protesting the conditions of their employment. Over their heads hung the threat of return to the institution. "I did not have to come back to the cottage until I get discharged from the farm, if the farmer don't like you, he send you back to the school, see" (Rowe, 2006). The war offered him escape, as it did for many. He was "glad when the war broke out", telling his employer that he intended to enlist. "'You can't! I'm not going to let you' he said. I said 'I'm going whether you like it or not.'" Early one morning he slipped away from the farm to a recruiting station and volunteered. After Japan entered the war in December 1941, his battalion shipped to Darwin, in the far north of Australia (Rowe, 2006). He recalled the repeated bombing raids inflicted by the Japanese: "Terrible. Damned terrible … Every night you'd get ready for bed, and the siren's going, you can't sleep after that, and they're dropping bombs all the time" (Manning, 2008, 119). Steven A. Gelb (2004) has pointed to the 'unplanned normalization of World War II' in the United States. For Ted, at least, the war provided the way out of institutions and into life in the community. After the war he married and found steady employment before retiring (Manning, 2008, 119).

In the first four decades of the twentieth century, fear of the feeble-minded prompted Victoria to establish a system intended to control those deemed mentally defective. In addition to the institutions through which Ted moved, in 1937 the Department of Mental Hygiene also established a Colony for Mental Defectives at Janefield on the outskirts of Melbourne. In 1939, after a second unsuccessful attempt 10 years earlier, a Mental Deficiency Act finally passed through parliament (Jones, 1999, 324–5). It was not immediately proclaimed, however, the Director of Mental Hygiene explaining that his Department was not yet able 'to accommodate the number of mentally retarded children whose supervision their parents desire the Department to undertake. There are fairly long waiting lists for both Travancore and Janefield, and until the latter Institution is further developed no benefit would accrue from putting the Act into operation' (Report of the Director of Mental Hygiene 1939, 36). However, construction of the first units for Janefield Farm Colony had begun (Report of Director of Mental Hygiene 1939, 3). These institutions were the inheritance with which the post-war era would have to contend.

'An unwanted inheritance from a less insightful past'

In April 1953 the *Herald* newspaper received a tip-off that a six-year-old 'mentally retarded' boy spent his days 'tied to a stake' in a Melbourne backyard. Investigating, journalist E.W. Tipping discovered that the boy's parents, shopkeepers, had restrained their son in an attempt to protect him while they worked. Theirs, Tipping explained, was an act of desperation, because their only alternative was to admit 'Michael' (not his real name) to Kew Cottages. It was not institutional care per se to which they objected, however, but the deplorable conditions into which past governments had allowed the Cottages to fall, recently exposed by the press (White, 1951, for example). Confronted by police and the media, Michael's mother declared that she would 'willingly send my child to an institution, but I will never send him to those terrible Kew Cottages as long as I live'. However, persuaded by the Cottages social worker that Michael 'could be happy and well looked after out at Kew', she relented (Tipping, 1953a; Scully, 2005). When Dr Eric Cunningham Dax, Chairman of the newly established Mental Hygiene Authority took Tipping to visit Michael at Kew, they found him, not by accident, in a recently renovated ward. Contrasting the bright, clean surrounds in Michael's ward with the primitive conditions elsewhere in the Cottages, Tipping argued they proved 'what can be done – even at Kew – if only adequate funds were available' and challenged the government to find the money to modernise the Cottages (Tipping, 1953b). Three days later, the *Herald* launched a public appeal to raise funds for improvements; the government subsequently pledged to match public donations pound for pound (*Herald*, 1953a; 1953b). Over two weeks, the appeal collected £47,798 (Edwards, 1972, 128; Lloyd, 1987, 25).

The tip-off which had alerted Tipping to the plight of Michael had in fact come from Dax, who cultivated relationships with the media as part of his campaign to reform the care of the mentally disordered in Victoria. As the then editor of the *Herald* later explained, the articles Tipping wrote used Michael's story as 'the peg for a greater theme: the Kew cottages must be transformed into places to which distracted parents would not be afraid to send their unfortunate children' (Edwards, 1972, 127; Robson, 2003, 278). The articles went further, promising that with proper funding the Cottages could become a place of hope, where mentally retarded children could be helped to live more fulfilling lives (Tipping, 1953b). Within two decades of Michael's admission, however, any role for institutions would be entirely rejected, and the Cottages viewed as 'an unwanted inheritance from a less insightful past' (Report on the Children's Cottages, 1979).

In June 1973, 20 years after the *Herald* reported Michael's story, another Melbourne newspaper began a campaign. In articles published under the ill-chosen title 'The Minus Children', the *Age* revealed a system of care 'on the brink of breakdown'. A government freeze on funds over the previous five years had created a severe shortage of institutional accommodation, leaving desperate parents waiting years for a place for their child, with little support in the meantime. Existing institutions grew increasingly overcrowded. Funding cutbacks had also hampered renovations, so that 'substandard accommodation', the legacy of past government neglect, still existed 'to a significant degree'. Reductions in the budget for new buildings were delaying the construction of a 500-bed training centre in Colac, 150 kilometres south-west of Melbourne. The Mental Health Authority proposed a five-year building blitz to provide 900 extra beds. Even this, experts believed, would not keep pace with 'projected needs' (Hills and Larkin, 1973).

Michael experienced all of this firsthand. When he was admitted in 1953 the Cottages were home to 414 residents (Report of the Mental Hygiene Authority 1953). By 1973, Michael was one of more than 900 residents. Wards intended to accommodate between 12 and 20 accommodated between 35 and 48 people (*Age*, 1973a). Two years after admission Michael was transferred to 'Little Pell'. Officially designated Ward 16A, Little Pell consisted of three corrugated iron huts salvaged from Camp Pell, a Second-World-War-era army camp. Little Pell was among the 'most deprived' of the Cottages' accommodation (Report of the Mental Hygiene Authority 1955, 57; Lloyd, 1987, 33; Manning, 2008, 90). Patrick Reed, admitted three years after Michael, recalled living there: "We were all in a kind of hut, and they had a big yard around it, and you had to stay in there all day ... [It was] real cold, and no heating" (Reed, 2006). As Corinne Manning (2008, 181) observes, 'For Michael, the benefits of being at the centre of the Tipping Appeal were short-lived'.

Responding to the *Age*, the Victorian premier, Rupert Hamer, 'promised a new deal for the minus children', pledging to reform special education and push ahead with the planned 'building and staffing of institutions' (*Age*, 1973b). But the government did little to fulfil these promises (*Age*, 1974a; 1974b; 1974c). In October 1974, the *Age* published a second series of articles 'which showed much of the situation was worse than before' (Larkin, 1974a; *Age*, 1974d). Given this 'gap between promise and performance, between provision and unrequited need', the *Age* questioned whether the government was 'capable of coping with this agonising human problem' and called on the premier to intervene (*Age*, 1974e). Two days later Hamer pledged to 'set up and head his own special committee to help the thousands of mentally retarded children in Victoria' (Larkin, 1974b). In 1977 the resulting Victorian Committee on Mental Retardation presented a report which asserted that normalisation should be 'the guiding principle in the provision of services' (Evans, 1977; Victorian Committee on Mental Retardation, 1977, 3–6). Its recommendation reflected increasing awareness and acceptance of normalisation in Victoria (Fox, 2003, 42).

With normalisation as its guiding principle, policy in Victoria shifted away from institutions towards services in the community (for example Houghton, 1978a; 1978b; 1978c). However, deinstitutionalisation proved a slow process. Beginning in 1981, when the government announced the closure of St Nicholas Hospital, it continued in fits and starts across the next three decades (Fox, 2003, 42–5). Kew Cottages was among the last to close. As other institutions were shuttered, the Cottages became more and more 'an anachronism, a relic of long-forgotten policies, retained by successive governments as a place of last resort for intellectually disabled men and women' (Fox, 2003, 37). How did the new policy direction affect people's lives? For some it provided an early escape. In 1981 Patrick Reed, who with Michael had endured Little Pell, was discharged from Kew and subsequently lived in hostels and independently, working to support himself (Manning, 2008, 122). Others, like Michael, remained confined for decades. How did normalisation impact their lives?

The Committee on Mental Retardation had emphasised that normalisation was 'both a process and a goal. Neither', it argued, 'should be regarded as absolute; service and practices [could] be ranked as more or less normalising *relative* [sic] to other services or past practices'. Normalisation within institutions was possible. It might:

> mean moving from the acceptance of bulk purchased, issued clothing to the personal selection of clothes from the store, to the purchase of clothes from community shops. The provision of ward-based educational programmes, attendance at outside day-education services, and progression to a community-based developmental home and separate community school can be successive stages in the normalisation process. (Victorian Committee on Mental Retardation, 1977, 5)

Attempts *were* made to 'normalise' the lives of residents at Kew (Fox, 2003, 39). Some dormitories, including the unit in which Michael was living, were partitioned into smaller living spaces. Communal clothing was dispensed with. Participation in day programmes and work placements increased (Fox, 2003, 39; Scully, 2005; Manning, 2008, 85–6, 97, 100–2). However, as was so often the case, government neglect and parsimony hampered efforts to make improvements. In October 1992 a 'fiercely neo-liberal' government swept to power. The cuts it inflicted 'resulted in a major cut to Kew's funding' (Fox, 2003, 37; Freckelton, 2005, 82–3). By 1995 the effects were so serious that the Kew Cottages Parents' Association made the decision to sue the government for failing to meet its obligation to provide services to the standard prescribed by the Intellectually Disabled Persons' Services Act 1986 (Godwin and Wade, 2007, 17; Manning, 2008, 155, 223). In April 1996, eight months after the Parents' Association instituted proceedings against the government, a fire in one of the residential units killed nine men. They, like Michael, had lived at Kew for many years, some for decades. The coronial inquest 'established beyond doubt' that the government had contributed to the men's deaths by failing to install a proper fire safety system (Fox, 2003, 37; Freckelton, 2005, 81–2). For disability advocates these deaths represented the tragic consequence of failing to fully implement normalisation and concomitant deinstitutionalisation (Freckelton, 2005).

The fire accelerated plans for deinstitutionalisation of Kew (Manning, 2008, 206, 209, 226). In 1999 the premier, Jeff Kennett, announced the intention to close the Cottages, confirmed by his successor, Steve Bracks, in 2001. Announcing the closure, Bracks 'expressed dismay at the "overcrowded and over-cramped dormitories" that he saw on his tour of the institution' (Soraghan, 2008a), revealing how limited were the results of attempts to normalise life there. In 2001, '480 people were living on the 27 acre site in just 16 residential units. Conditions were inadequate and overcrowded … there were many instances of four or five residents sharing a bedroom that was in effect a partitioned dormitory' (Intellectual Disability Review Panel, 2007, 49). Over the next seven years, most residents moved from the Cottages into small group homes in the community. On 20 April 2008, 120 years after opening, the last 100 residents moved into houses built as part of a new suburb developed on the site (Soraghan, 2008b). Michael's family hoped that he would stay on the redeveloped site, his sister Mary arguing that he had a right to do so: "he's done a lot for Kew, in his way, by the Tipping Appeal. It has been his home for 50 years, why can't it be his home for the rest of his life?" (Scully,

2005). However, after 52 years there, Michael moved instead into a community house.

Conclusion

The life histories in this chapter reveal that in the nexus between policy and practice, the impact on people's lives could prove paradoxical. When policy emphasised segregation, Ted Rowe was able to find his way back to life in the community. Michael, in contrast, lived for decades in an institution as policy increasingly emphasised normalisation and deinstitutionalisation. He, along with thousands of others, was living out the legacy of the previous era. Their stories suggest that the ways in which policy impacts on people's lives may not always be what we expect.

Acknowledgement

The author would like to thank Dr Janet Butler for her helpful comments on an earlier version of this chapter.

References

Age (1934) 'Women citizens: visit to Travancore', 27 June, p 13.

Age (1936) 'Work at Travancore', 20 November, p 24.

Age (1973a) 'The Minus Children: Part Four', 14 June, *The Minus Children: A series of articles reprinted from The Age*, Melbourne, 1974, np.

Age (1973b) 'Retarded get new education deal', 23 June, *The Minus Children: A series of articles reprinted from The Age*, Melbourne, 1974, np.

Age (1974a) 'All's quiet: Colin's dead', 23 January, *The Minus Children: A series of articles reprinted from The Age*, Melbourne, 1974, np.

Age (1974b) 'Govt and the Minus Children', 24 January, *The Minus Children: A series of articles reprinted from The Age*, Melbourne, 1974, np.

Age (1974c) 'Minus Children, minus policies', 7 February, in *The Minus Children: A series of articles reprinted from The Age*, Melbourne, 1974, np.

Age (1974d) 'The Minus Children revisited: part two', 11 October, in *The Minus Children: A series of articles reprinted from The Age*, Melbourne, 1974, np.

Age (1974e) 'Still the Minus Children wait', 14 October, in *The Minus Children: A series of articles reprinted from The Age*, Melbourne, 1974, np.

Argyle, S. (1926) *Victorian parliamentary debates*, vol 127, 6 October, pp 1851–67.

Argyle, S. (1929) *Victorian parliamentary debates*, vol 173, 13 August, p 800.

Earl, D. (2018) 'Australian histories of intellectual disabilities', in R. Hanes, I. Brown and N.E. Hansen (eds) *The Routledge history of disability*, Oxford and New York: Routledge, pp 308–19.

Edwards, C. (1972) *The editor regrets*, Melbourne: Hill of Content.

Fishbourne, J.W.Y. (1913) 'The segregation of the epileptic and feeble-minded', in Australasian Medical Congress (formerly the Intercolonial Medical Congress of Australasia), *Transactions of the ninth session held in Sydney, New South Wales, September 1911*, Sydney: William Applegate Gullick, Government Printer, pp 885–91.

Fox, C. (2003) 'Debating deinstitutionalisation: the fire at Kew Cottages in 1996 and the idea of community', *Health and History*, 5(2), 37–59.

Freckelton, I. (2005) 'Institutional death: the coronial inquest into the deaths of nine men with intellectual disabilities', in K. Johnson and R. Traustadóttir (eds) *Deinstitutionalization and people with intellectual disabilities: In and out of institutions*, London and Philadelphia: Jessica Kingsley Publishers, pp 76–85.

Gelb, S.A. (2004) '"Mental deficients" fighting fascism: the unplanned normalization of WWII' in S. Noll and J.W. Trent (eds) *Mental retardation in America: A historical reader*, New York and London: New York University Press, pp 308–21.

Godwin, L. and Wade, C. (2007) *Kew Cottages Parents' Association: The first fifty years 1957 to 2007*, Melbourne: Kew Cottages Parents' Association.

Herald (1953a) 'Many give to *Herald* appeal', 11 April, p 1.

Herald (1953b) 'Govt. gives £ for £', 14 April, p 1.

Hills, B. and Larkin, J. (1973) 'Pity the retarded, ours is the shame', *Age*, 11 June, in *The Minus Children: A series of articles reprinted from The Age*, Melbourne (1974).

Intellectual Disability Review Panel (2007) *A right to be heard: IDRP: 1987-2007*, Melbourne, Intellectual Disability Review Panel.

Jones, R. (1999) 'The master potter and the rejected pots: eugenic legislation in Victoria, 1918–1939', *Australian Historical Studies*, 30(113), 319–42.

Larkin, J. (1974a) 'The Minus Children revisited', 10 October, in *The Minus Children: A series of articles reprinted from The Age*, Melbourne, 1974, np.

Larkin, J. (1974b) 'Premier will champion our retarded children', *Age*, 17 October, in *The Minus Children: A series of articles reprinted from The Age*, Melbourne, 1974, np.

Lewis, J. (1989) 'Removing the grit: the development of special education in Victoria 1887–1947', PhD, LaTrobe University.

Lloyd, A. (1987) *Payment by results: Kew Cottages' first 100 years 1887–1987*, Melbourne: Kew Cottages and St Nicholas Parents' Association.

Manning, C. (2008) *Bye-Bye Charlie: Stories from the vanishing world of Kew Cottages*, Sydney: UNSW Press.

Manning, C. (2010) '"My memory's back!" Inclusive learning disability research using ethics, oral history and digital storytelling', *British Journal of Learning Disabilities*, 38(3), 160–7.

Monk, L. and Manning, C. (2012) 'Exploring patient experience in an Australian institution for children with learning disabilities, 1887–1933', in A. Borsay and P. Dale (eds) *Disabled children: Contested caring, 1850–1979*, London: Pickering and Chatto, pp 87–102.

Reed, P. (2006) Interview with Manning, C., Kew Cottages History Project Archive, La Trobe University.

Report of the Director of Mental Hygiene 1939 (1940) *Victorian parliamentary papers*, vol I.

Report of the Director of Mental Hygiene 1941 (1942–3) *Victorian parliamentary papers*, vol I.

Report of the Inspector-General of the Insane 1925 (1927) *Victorian parliamentary papers*, vol II.

Report of the Inspector-General of the Insane 1926 (1927) *Victorian parliamentary papers*, vol II.

Report of the Inspector-General of the Insane (Director of Mental Hygiene) 1933 (1935) *Victorian parliamentary papers*, vol I.

Report of the Mental Hygiene Authority 1953 (1954–55) *Victorian parliamentary papers*, vol 3.

Report of the Mental Hygiene Authority 1955 (1955–56) *Victorian parliamentary papers*, vol 2.

Robson, B. (2003) '"He made us feel special": Eric Cunningham Dax, Edith Pardy and the reform of mental health services in Victoria, 1950s and 1960s', *Australian Historical Studies*, 34 (122), 270-89.

Rowe, E. (2006) Interview with Manning, C., Kew Cottages History Project Archive, La Trobe University.

Scully, M. (2005) Interview with Manning, C., Kew Cottages History Project Archive, La Trobe University.

Soraghan, K. (2008a) 'The Kew Redevelopment … looking back through *Kew News*', *Kew News*, May 2008, pp 6-7.

Soraghan, K. (2008b) 'An era ends, and a new way of life begins', *Kew News*, May 2008, p 1.

Tipping, E.W. (1953a) 'The story of 6-year-old-Michael who was tied to a stake', *Herald*, 6 April.

Tipping, E.W. (1953b) 'Why Michael has not tried to run away', *Herald*, 7 April.

Victorian Committee on Mental Retardation (1977) *Report of the Victorian Committee on Mental Retardation: Report to the premier of Victoria, August 1977*, Melbourne: Government Printer.

White, O. (1951) 'Their misery is our shame', *Herald*, 28 August, p 4.

Archival material

Department of Human Services, Victoria Archives, A/S 92/184/4, Kew Cottages file, Edward Rowe.

Evans, J.L. to Houghton, W.V. (1977) PROV, VPRS 6345/P0, Unit 516, File 1908, Premier's Committee on Mental Retardation, 3 October.

Houghton, W.V. to Wragg, H. (1978a) PROV, VPRS 6345/P0, Box 480, File 1644 Part 4, 17 January.

Houghton, W.V. (1978b) Recommendation to cabinet for implementation of policies in mental retardation, PROV, VPRS 6344/P1, Box 21, File 60/32 Part 2, 21 September.

Houghton, W.V. to Temby, E. (1978c) PROV, VPRS 6345/P0, Box 480, File 1644 Part 4, 16 October.

National Archives of Australia: B884, V240186, Rowe, Edward.

PROV (Public Record Office Victoria), VPRS 7491/P1 Travancore Special School Records, History Card.

PROV, VPRS 7565/P1 Admission Warrants, Male and Female Patients, Unit 7.

Report on the Children's Cottages (1979) PROV, VPRS 6345/P0, Unit 368, File Z/657 Part II.

TWO

Tracing the historical and ideological roots of services for people with intellectual disabilities in Austria

Gertraud Kremsner, Oliver Koenig and Tobias Buchner

Setting the scene: discovering the past – dismantling the present

This chapter focuses on how historical and contemporary influences have affected the development of policy and practice of services for people with intellectual disabilities in Austria. We start with an exploration of the production and development of eugenic discourses. We show how these discourses were explicitly adopted by institutions at the beginning of the twentieth century, reached their height during the Nazi regime, but, even though officially condemned, influenced service provision after 1945 through both ideological and personal continuities. In the post-war era, most people with intellectual disabilities who did not live with their families had to live in psychiatric hospitals or large Christian or state-run institutions. Parent-led organisations, which were developing from the mid-1960s, led to the first significant change in quality of services for persons with intellectual disabilities. In the late 1970s, discourses around normalisation and integration swept over from Scandinavia, impacting strongly on the field. In the following two decades, deinstitutionalisation programmes were implemented, which led to a 'life in the community' for most former inmates of psychiatric wards. However, these programmes mostly focused on psychiatric hospitals, leaving other large institutional settings untouched, thus the term 'de-hospitalisation' seems more appropriate than deinstitutionalisation. The chapter closes by indicating that – despite several policy changes and efforts to create a more personalised system of care since the 2000s – the institutional system of service provision contains serious problems. We point to the continuing influence of eugenic discourses and practices, and to illustrate the impact of disabling ideologies and practices, we feature some abbreviated life stories.

The historical and ideological roots of institutionalisation

Unfolding the history of institutionalisation in Austria is – just as in other countries – rather complex; a distinct starting point and single line of development cannot be identified. However, the foundation of the so-called Viennese 'tower of fools' in 1784, which is considered to be the first modern European psychiatric hospital, marks an important date for the history of psychiatric care in Austria (Ledebur, 2015).

In the course of the nineteenth century, reformist institutions were founded for persons with intellectual disabilities (eg the foundation of 'Levana' by Georgens and Deinhardt in 1854). These charitable institutions, most with a confessional background, continue to the present day to stand as milestones, with a large number of historical sources that have been researched extensively. By contrast, little is known about 'regular', large-scale accommodation at that time. While adults with intellectual disabilities from wealthy and bourgeois families were incarcerated in institutions for 'idiots' or 'cretins' (where they were basically taken into custody), particularly in the first half of the 19th century, prisons, poorhouses and asylums served as institutions for family members of the majority of the underprivileged population (Droste, 1999) – at a time when Social Darwinism increasingly became popular (reaching full bloom by the end of the nineteenth century). In the same era, psychiatry became an independent medical discipline and thus scientific and medical interest in 'feeble-mindedness' increased dramatically (Droste, 1999). This went hand in hand with omnipotent fantasies of the medical profession being able to cure and heal everyone (Strachota, 2002). Due to the profound transformation of economic and political conditions in the second half of the nineteenth century – workers were exploited to the maximum and left with poor medical and social care (Häßler and Häßler, 2005) – the previously envisaged differentiation in accommodation for 'idiots' on the one hand and 'lunatics' on the other could not be met (Droste, 1999). As a result, most persons with intellectual disabilities were sent to asylums which increased rapidly in numbers in the second half of the nineteenth century (Schmidt, 1993).

Institutionalisation took on new dimensions with the foundation of clinical psychiatry – modern asylums with the structure of a hospital – in the beginning of the twentieth century. Initially planned as modern institutions with the aim to not only avoid restrictive methods and coercive treatment but also to offer therapy and occupation, these clinics soon turned into 'overcrowded Ghettos in which idiots, alcoholics, lunatics, geriatric patients, suicidal and all other deviant persons'[1] (Schmidt, 1993, 46; own translation) were kept locked up side by side. These clinics collaborated closely with youth welfare institutions – which led to many children and youngsters being sent to psychiatric hospitals, and remaining there after reaching the legal age of adulthood. In Eastern Austria, the psychiatric clinics 'Am Steinhof' in Vienna (founded 1907) and 'Gugging' in Lower Austria (founded 1885) were explicitly assigned to accommodate adults as well as children with intellectual disabilities in large numbers (Ledebur, 2015). More or less at the same time, eugenic discourses provided pseudo-scientific legitimation: Alfred Plötz's book *Grundlinien einer Rassenhygiene* (*Baselines of Race Hygiene*) was published in 1895 and gained great popularity, in the aftermath of the global economic crisis in 1908 when media openly discussed the usefulness of 'unproductive eaters' (Häßler and Häßler, 2005).

After the outbreak of the First World War, living conditions in asylums changed dramatically. This was initially evident through a significant decrease in staff members, many of whom had been called to military service (Ledebur, 2015), and was boosted by an influx of patients with war-induced trauma. By 1916, the mortality rate in psychiatric clinics reached its peak due to poor supplies during the war (Ledebur, 2015), which had led to a reduction of rations particularly for persons with intellectual disabilities (Häßler and Häßler, 2005). With the 'Imperial Incapacitation Order' (RGBl. Nr. 207), admission to psychiatric clinics was regulated by law for the first time in 1916 and remained in force as applicable law for legal guardianship until 1984.

After the First World War, psychiatric institutions in Austria lost their last spark of reformist attempts and turned into camps – due to massive homelessness, high unemployment and inflation (Ledebur, 2015). Although some 'special units' for persons with intellectual disabilities were founded, their 'accommodation' was characterised by plain drug administration (Plangger and Schönwiese, 2010), accompanied by modern forms of 'treatment' such as insulin-, malaria- or other invasive shock therapies (Heiss, 2015). Simultaneously, the collapse of the Austrian Empire in 1918 led to changes in administration, which affected psychiatric clinics. Of particular relevance are Julius Tandler's reforms. He introduced a modern system of health care (including predecessors of social psychiatry), youth welfare and care for the poor (Sieder, 2014) – systems which were designed to work closely with each other. Psychiatric diagnoses not only formed the basis for psychiatric admissions but also for assigning children and youngsters to children's homes (Sieder, 2014). Less well-known is the rooting of these reforms in eugenic and utilitarian discourses with the aim of achieving a healthy and productive 'body of the people' ('Volkskörper'), for whom inmates of psychiatric hospitals and those sent to children's homes were seen as an economic burden. Tandler wanted to 'nip bodily and mental inferiority in the bud'[2] (Ledebur, 2015, 213; own translation). At the same time, in 1920, Binding and Hoche published their book *Allowing the Elimination of Life Unworthy of Living (Die Freigabe der Vernichtung lebensunwerten Lebens)*, which gained high popularity in Austria. Amplified by the stock market crash in 1929, utilitarian and eugenic considerations spread massively, by media finding multiple examples of setting off costs of 'inferior persons' against 'healthy families' (Häßler and Häßler, 2005). In the course of the next decade, these considerations and attitudes led to the darkest chapter in Austrian (disability) history: National Socialism.

The mass elimination programme of 'unworthy' life under National Socialism

As we have shown, National Socialism in Austria didn't appear from nowhere. Instead, 'all ingredients were already composed' (Ralser, 2014, 140; own translation) long before Austria was affiliated to Nazi-Germany. Social Darwinist and eugenic discourses culminated in the 'Law for the Prevention of Offspring with Hereditary Diseases', which came into force in 1933 in Germany and – with a slight delay after the Anschluss – in 1940 in Austria (Reichsgesetzblatt, 1939). With this law, thousands of so-called 'hereditarily diseased persons' had to undergo forced sterilisation; including large numbers of persons with intellectual disabilities (Mattner, 2000).

In 1939, a secret circular letter obliged midwives and physicians to report 'malformed and idiotic' new-born babies (Czech, 2014), which marked the beginning of euthanasia. File records of reported children were sent to reviewers, who decided upon life or – in most cases – death in one of the specifically created 'special units for children' ('Kinderfachabteilungen'). Parents were forced to give their consent: if they refused, they lost custody of their children (Mattner, 2000). In most cases, children died from an overdose of Luminal, which led to pneumonia and thus – following the cynical logic of National Socialists – to 'natural death' (Biewer, 2009). Between 1939 and 1945 nearly 5,000 children were killed in that manner (Czech, 2014). With similar administrative procedure and under strictest secrecy, 'Aktion T4' came into force on 2 September 1939, which aimed at annihilating adults with intellectual disabilities (Häßler and Häßler, 2005). Persons who were 'allowed for elimination' (see Binding and Hoche, 1920) were sent to gas chambers at five locations in Germany, but also to Hartheim in Upper Austria. Around 100,000 persons were systematically killed in those 'institutions', among them 18,269 in Austrian territory at Hartheim (Mattner, 2000). Despite utmost secrecy, 'Aktion T4' was officially stopped in 1941 as a result of massive and mostly uncoordinated civil protest stemming from different sources. Whilst protest from the Catholic Church was claimed to have stopped official euthanasia, members of the underground communist party as well as allied forces circulated leaflets scandalising the mass murder. Among the different forms of resistance, parental activism to protect one's own children from deportation was the most organised. There were both organised rallies in front of 'Am Steinhof' following the first deportations, and letters to the 'Reichsinnenministerium' (Ministry of the Interior). However, these efforts couldn't stop 'wild euthanasia' – in particular through food deprivation and medication overdose in psychiatric clinics. An estimated 185,000 victims were killed (Häßler and Häßler, 2005). These atrocities marked the culmination of societal attitudes and opinions initiated long before the takeover of the Nazi regime: '[those] who were economically not exploitable were eradicated; those who were capable of work were allowed to survive' (Weiss, 1978, 55). Besides psychiatric clinics and other medical institutions, church-run nursing homes and a 'pedagogy which could not bear to deal with those persons who were said to lack abilities'[3] (Malina, 2007, 103) played a key role in this system of annihilation.

The psychiatric clinic 'Am Steinhof' serves as a good example of personal and 'professional' continuities after the end of the Nazi regime. The clinics' pavilions 15 and 17 had served as killing institutions. These pavilions seamlessly continued to 'accommodate' persons with intellectual disabilities up until the (late) 1990s (Mayrhofer et al, 2017). After the Second World War, most of the same personnel continued to work in these units. Heinrich Gross, one of the key physicians of the pavilions during the Nazi regime, did not only continue to work in the clinic, but also developed his career long after the war on the basis of brain slices of nearly 600 former inmates who had been killed in the pavilions (Czech, 2002). Similar continuities can be found in other psychiatric hospitals in Austria after 1945 as many protagonists returned to their (leading) positions in psychiatric hospitals (Berger, 1996). Irma's story documents both the eugenic cruelties of the Nazi regime and post-war efforts to mask the continuities both on a personnel and ideological level.

Irma's story

This story is taken from the documentary 'My sister Irma', in which Antje Kosemund investigates the story of her sister Irma, who was incarcerated in Hamburg, then deported to the 'Spiegelgrund' clinic in Vienna where she was murdered in 1944 (Kosemund, 2005).

Irma was born on 20 January 1933 in Hamburg, the seventh of 12 siblings. In the same year their father, an active member of the antifascist labour movement was arrested by the Gestapo and subsequently lost his job. Even though confronted with hunger, Antje recalls happy childhood memories with her sister Irma. It soon became obvious that Irma's development was delayed. A neighbour denounced the family, reporting on a child in the family who seemed not 'normal'. After Irma's mother refused to consult an officer of the family welfare service, a warrant was issued for Irma to be presented to a psychiatrist. The assessment read: 'a completely idiotic child, flat occiput, hair growth that reaches far on the forehead, bumps on the forehead, broad jaw'. These descriptions did not match Irma's actual appearance documented on photographs depicting a pretty girl with a fringe haircut and big brown eyes. Pressured by the welfare service, the parents agreed to send her to the 'Alsterdorfer Anstalten', an asylum for children and adults with disabilities. With Irma's disappearance, she soon was lost from family memory. More than 40 years later, in 1983, Antje was re-confronted with the death of her sister, when she accidentally found Irma's certificate of death. Antje immediately noticed something was not right and consulted a historian who encouraged her to continue investigations. She got hold of a list of children who had been deported from Alsterdorf to 'Am Steinhof', which contained Irma's name. This discovery led her to write letters to representatives of these two institutions, inquiring further information about her sister. Alsterdorf sent copies of her sister's patient file, revealing the suffering of a child who had been isolated, had lost most of her abilities and frequently was strapped to bed when she tried to resist mistreatment. All she received from Vienna was an excuse that her sister's patient files must have been lost in the turmoil of war and that her remains had been buried in an anonymous mass grave. Since Antje had no reason then to distrust the information received she ended her investigations, until 12 years later (in 1995) she saw a TV documentary about the 'brain-chamber', a room in the cellar of the department of pathology at 'Am Steinhof'. In this chamber medical preparations of euthanasia victims were being stored. When she found out that her sister's brain was also stored there, Antje started a year-long correspondence, which bears well-documented witness to unwillingness on the part of official bodies in Austria to address this issue. It required another act of boldness on the part of Antje to directly address the Austrian president and chancellor, as well as subsequent media interest, until in 1996 Irma's remains, alongside those of 12 other former inmates were sent back to Hamburg and buried in a dignified memorial ceremony. Six years later in 2002, after the brain-chamber had been officially closed and the remains of more than 800 people buried, Antje was informed that Irma's files had reappeared. They had been found in a locked cabinet and contained the full documentations of Irma as well as five other former inmates, all of whom had relatives who, many years after the war, had started to inquire about the circumstances of their deaths. It was only then that Antje was able to read about the full horrors of what had happened to her sister, and that Professor Gross had continued to work on her sister's tissue up until 1956, when the last entry in her records was made. Antje Kosemund was awarded the German Federal Cross of Merit in 2013.

After 1945: Continuities and resistance, de-hospitalisation and deinstitutionalisation

As shown in Irma's story, the end of the National Socialist regime did not lead to a fundamental reorientation – on the contrary, (eugenic) concepts and structures from the inter-war years were re-established (Plangger and Schönwiese, 2010), with personnel educated and/or employed during National Socialism. 'After 1945, psychiatric care didn't change a lot compared to the inter-war years. Institutions, emptied by fascist actions, were restocked without any kind of reform'[4] (Weiss, 1978, 55; own translation). Even though mass murder was stopped, the associated attitudes did not disappear. Psychiatric hospitals and children's homes – still the only institutions accommodating persons with intellectual disabilities – took on the role of 'the extended arm of society in terms of excluding and isolating "deviant" individuals'[5] (Schmidt, 1993, 48). Schönwiese (2013) describes how after only a short period of formal distancing from the cruelties of National Socialism the institutional and psychiatric care system quickly bounced back to a mode of 'business as usual', and tried to market a 'humanised' institutional and psychiatric care model.

Eugenic discourses still played a role. Andreas Rett's work serves as an example. Although not accused of taking part in any of the death institutions, Rett's proximity to National Socialism can be reconstructed (Schönwiese, 2012). In 1968, he published an article based on the already mentioned brain slices, together with Heinrich Gross (see above). As a famous psychiatrist – he was the first to describe 'Rett's Syndrome' – he was considered to be *the* expert in intellectual disabilities in Austria until his death in 1997. Rett openly acknowledged his eugenic approach in several publications and lectures, but first and foremost by his demand for the forced sterilisation of women with intellectual disabilities, which was implemented for an uncountable number of women (Zemp and Pircher, 1996). This practice was legally in force until 2001 (Schönwiese, 2012). It was also Rett who – along with others – publicly called for 'indicated abortion' due to eugenic reasons and who linked the newly passed law to permit (late) abortion to 'early care measures': 'How many families do we have – do I know personally – in which we knew with 100% certainty that every child will be ill. Nevertheless, abortion was not allowed to be executed. I truly believe that [with the new law] a health policy has been implemented which will have a real preventive effect on the area of disability and will be of enormous significance'[6] (Rett, in JG SPÖ NÖ 1980, 7).

Resistance to the dominating, and until the late 1950s the only available, institutional and psychiatric care model took different shapes. One generative spark for the transition towards a post- or rather adjunct service form next to the institutional and psychiatric care model (although governed by guiding medical and deficit-based assumptions) came directly from parents who lobbied for the implementation of rehabilitation-oriented services as an alternative to placement in institutions from the 1960s. Coming from a labour welfare tradition and aimed mostly at supporting youth who, after the demolitions of the Second World War, had only few opportunities to receive vocational training, the organisation 'Jugend am Werk' ('Youth at work') opened the first sheltered workshops for disabled adults, which also became the guiding example for the newly established parent-led 'Lebenshilfe' organisations with a primary orientation towards occupation, therapeutic development and security. The first accommodation services were established in 1961 (Lebenshilfe Vienna) and 1965 (Jugend am Werk) (Kremsner, 2017). Due to growing pressure from parents and following field visits to Sweden, 'Lebenshilfe' established group homes for 24 inhabitants as a new standard for supported accommodation, often combined with a sheltered workshop 'under one roof'. These new structures meant, compared to the huge institutions, an increase in quality of life. However, they still had to be considered as institutions. Care followed an individualistic model of disability and included a clear hierarchy between 'users' and 'caretakers'. Mostly established with a parental board structure, there was no formal representation of the interests of service users who had little say over aspects governing their daily life. Personnel and ideological continuities also affected these organisations, with Andreas Rett, who offered regular consultancy, being referred to as one of the 'founding fathers'. He became chairman of the 'Federal Advisory Committee for the Disabled' in 1976 to help establish more organisations (Schönwiese, 2012).

Parent-led organisations continued to grow steadily from the 1970s onwards, and together with large institutions characterised available service options until the late 1980s and early 1990s.

Critiques of the practices of large institutions were, by then, not only raised by parents but also by social movements[7] who took on a leading role for demanding change. The first locally organised independent living organisations played a key role. Under the heading 'Who wants to live in an institution?', proponents of this movement questioned paternalistic, disempowering living conditions through a range of activism, including radical interventions in public spaces from the late 1960s until the present day.[8] However, persons with intellectual disabilities had no or only little impact on this movement. Their living conditions were noticed by members of the movement, but not prioritised.

Civil protest by the international and locally growing anti-psychiatric and normalisation movements led to the first scientific study of the living conditions of residents in psychiatric hospitals (Forster and Pelikan, 1978) and caused considerable pressure on political decision makers in Austria. Vienna was the first federal state to react by developing a strategic plan in 1979, which aimed at moving persons out of psychiatric hospitals (Buchner, 2009). Even though persons with intellectual disabilities were also 'living' there in large numbers, their situation was only mentioned in passing (Kremsner, 2017). Only in 1986 the 'Declaration of Strategies for the Care of Disabled Persons' was adopted in Vienna, which aimed at founding 1,000 residential places in 10 years (Berger, 1996). This marked the starting point of the first wave of countrywide efforts of deinstitutionalisation (in official terminology), in practice de-hospitalisation, beginning in the mid 1980s, albeit to varying degrees. It was similar to other European countries in privileging persons labelled as having mild intellectual disabilities.

The scope of the task and subsequent emergence of a new type of professionally driven organisations was massively increased when a new series of press disclosures, most of them stemming from social movement activists and/or investigative journalists, gave rise to a new and important policy of deinstitutionalisation (focused only on psychiatric hospitals). In January 1991, the national 'Law on the Placement of Persons in Psychiatric Hospitals' (Unterbringungsgesetz

1990) came into force. According to this new law, psychiatric hospitals were not regarded as places of residence for people with intellectual disabilities, which marked the need for de-hospitalisation. Gerhard's story is about living in a psychiatric hospital and being part of the de-hospitalisation programme.

Gerhard's story

This story is taken from a Life History Research Project, in which former inmates who had lived in psychiatric hospitals in Vienna told their story (Westermann and Buchner, 2008).

Gerhard was born in 1973. At age five, he fell out of the window of his family's flat and suffered a serious head injury. After brain surgery, he was diagnosed as having an intellectual impairment and was sent to the children's ward of a psychiatric hospital, where he lived for the next few years. He went to a small special school, located at the hospital. Gerhard remembers a lot of conflicts with the other children living at the ward, but also a very caring relationship with a nurse he called 'auntie'. After a few years, the children's ward closed and Gerhard was sent to Pavillon 15, the children's ward of the psychiatric hospital 'Baumgartner Höhe' which also was part of the 'Spiegelgrund' (see 'Irma's story' above). There, he went through a very bad time: "Pavillon 15 was a horror trip. They kept giving me injections to keep me calm. That was the main aim of the caretakers: keeping me calm. They always gave me pills. They gave me only the strong ones [...] But not just once, I had to take them on a regular basis. Sometimes, they put me in a straitjacket and threw me in a cage bed which caused me bruises. Being in a straitjacket was terrible. I had the feeling I was going to choke, I could hardly breathe. But I was not the only one. They gave these injections to all of us. Nurses were our caretakers. They were very strict and unfriendly" (Westermann and Buchner, 2008, 129).

After some years, Gerhard was moved into Pavillon 17, which, as part of the Viennese de-hospitalisation programme, was dedicated to 'training' inmates to adapt to society. In the new pavilion, walls were coloured and Gerhard got his own room on the ground floor. However, Gerhard was sedated on a regular basis.

In 1993, Gerhard was moved into a small flat, where he was supported by a community support team for several hours a week. Gerhard considers this as a turning point, as it enabled him to lead his life more in a way as he wants it. However, living in the community was not easy in the beginning. Gerhard's new neighbours complained that they now 'had to live with a disabled guy in one house' and some youths harassed him. But Gerhard also made new friends in his neighbourhood, with whom he went to parks and restaurants. Looking back, Gerhard concludes on his life in the community: "There were good times and there were bad times."

In Gerhard's story, we can see how the pressure for deinstitutionalisation and 'normalisation' led to a differentiation of living arrangements, based on the Austrian model of so-called community-based living, such as residential houses, shared flats or group homes, and supported living in single or double flats (Buchner, 2009). The growing diversity of service offerings also forced the continuing adaptation of parental organisations from the early 1990s onwards, which slowly reorganised and tried to establish more person-centred ways of support. However, as we show with Kathi's story, the implementation of the Austrian model of community-based living includes strongly institutionalised practices.

Kathi's story

Kathi was one of the co-researchers in the project 'From confining the excluded to excluding the confined: biographical experiences from people with intellectual disabilities' (Kremsner, 2017).

Born in 1974, Kathi grew up in a tiny village and went to kindergarten there, before local authorities decided to send her to a special kindergarten due to her physical impairment. After one year in a regular secondary school, she was sent to a special boarding school at age 11. This transition marked the starting point for an institutional career: after finishing special school, she was sent to job training for persons with disabilities in Vienna which was linked to a group home. Kathi never worked at the job she was trained for but was sent to a sheltered workshop instead. At the age of 20, she had a miscarriage. Kathi recalls that both parents and caretakers at the group home 'applauded and were happy' that she lost the baby, while she felt 'like shit' (K4, in Kremsner, 2017, 187). Nevertheless, she stayed there for the next 13 years, before she moved to the group home in which she still lives. Today, Kathi doesn't feel 'intellectually disabled', although people around her regularly tell her she is. What makes her feel disabled is the type of care she experiences: "I live with full time care. This means that whenever I say I have to fart, all staff members run to me"[9] (K7, in Kremsner, 2017, 187). She doesn't want to live with other people and hates to be dependent on caretakers' moods. To sum up her experiences with institutional life, she says: "I feel crappy,

I feel crappy in this bitch-ass-group home. One should never send kids to this place. Because I live right here and exactly know how kids should be treated. One should never do that to kids deliberately"[10] (K2, in Kremsner, 2017, 188).

As one can see, besides the institutionalised 'service provision', Kathi's story also illustrates that eugenic discourses continue to impact on the field of services for persons with intellectual disabilities. The applause for the miscarriage stands as an example of the continuity of eugenic ideologies in Austria.

The current state: stagnation and continuity

Over the last decade, a lot of service providers have – in part due to the implementation of the CRPD (Convention on the Rights of Persons with Disabilities) – made serious efforts to modify their style of service provision and tried to shape support more according to the needs of users. Many Austrian federal states have stopped investing money in the re-creation of large residential facilities and prefer decentralised models with a decoupling of tenancy and support provision. However, serious problems still remain. First of all, some large-scale institutions were left untouched and still exist (Monitoringausschuss, 2017). Regimes of institutional care with more than 100 persons living and working in the same place still exist in five out of nine Austrian provinces and strategies for permanent deinstitutionalisation are not in place. Furthermore, even where de-hospitalisation has been officially considered complete, some persons with intellectual disabilities still have to live for long periods in psychiatric clinics (Kremsner, 2017). As indicated in Kathi's story, some of the practice in the field can be characterised as institutionalised, disempowering, dehumanising and based on the individual model of disability. In addition, persons who are labelled as persons with a 'severe impairment' seem to live mostly in large group homes with more than 12 persons or in institutions (Monitoringausschuss, 2017). Personal assistance is only available for a handful of persons with intellectual disabilities (Buchner, 2018). In many cases, contemporary large institutions mask themselves under progressive terminology whilst keeping the assumption alive that for some people an institution is the best place to live. Growing pressure on public households, demands for accountability and transparency in the use of public funds, coupled with new managerial discourses both in the running of services and public administration, are happening within a worrying political and societal drift to the far right. The erosion of societal solidarity contributes to the continuation and prolongation of both subtle and explicit eugenic mind-sets, discourses and practices.

In their position paper on bio-politics the umbrella organisation of independent living organisations (SLIÖ 2014) uses the term 'Euthanasia of everyday life' to signify the multitude of deliberate social and structural discriminations disabled people face on a day-to-day basis. Apart from that, both the entry and exit points of life are and have been subject to eugenic practices and discourses. In a parliamentary debate in December 2014, following a new legislative proposal on preimplantation diagnostics, former minister of health Sabine Oberhauser emphasised that the Austrian government is not planning to abolish the legal practice of 'eugenic indication', which means that a (most likely) impaired foetus can be aborted up to birth (Austrian Parliament, 2014). Concerning the end of life, SLIÖ warns about the inherent danger in replacing the needed societal debate around independent living and self-determination with a debate around independent dying and assisted suicide where, at regular intervals and prolonged through often uncritical media coverage, disabled life is often portrayed as life less worth living.

Notes

[1] Original quote: '[Psychiatrien verkommen zu] völlig überbelegten Gettos, in denen neben "Schwachsinnigen" Alkoholiker, psychisch Kranke, geriatrische Patienten, Suizidgefährdete und alle irgendwie auffällig gewordenen Normabweichler angehalten wurden' (Schmidt, 1993, 46).

[2] Original quote: '"körperliche und geistige Minderwertigkeit" (…), [sollten], so sein Programm, bereits im Keim erstickt werden' (Ledebur, 2015, 213).

[3] Original quote: 'In unheilvoller Allianz mit einer Pädagogik, die es nicht ertragen konnte, mit Schwachen, Kranken und angeblich nicht "Leistungsfähigen" umzugehen' (Malina, 2007, 103).

[4] Original quote: 'Nach 1945 änderte sich im Bereich der psychiatrischen Versorgung im Vergleich zur Vorkriegszeit zunächst nicht allzu viel. Die durch die faschistischen Maßnahmen geleerten Anstalten wurden wieder aufgefüllt, ohne daß es zu Reformen irgendwelcher Art gekommen wäre' (Weiss, 1978, 55).

[5] Original quote: Die Rolle der Psychiatrie erfüllt die Funktion eines 'verlängerten Armes der Gesellschaft bei der Ausgrenzung und Isolierung von "abweichenden" Individuen' (Schmidt, 1993, 48f.).

[6] Original quote: 'Wie viele Familien haben wir – kenne ich persönlich – wo man mit hundertprozentiger Sicherheit wusste, jedes weitere Kind wird

krank werden, und trotzdem ist es nicht möglich, Schwangerschaftsabbrüche durchzuführen. Ich glaube also, dass hier eine gesundheitspolitische Aktion, Aktivität gesetzt wurde, die auf dem Gebiet der Behinderung echt prophylaktische Wirkung hat und von enormer Bedeutung ist' (Rett, in JG SPÖ NÖ 1980, 7).

[7] Due to limited space, civil movements leading to a change in youth welfare cannot be described intensively here, but at least have to be mentioned. Parallel to the anti-psychiatric movement of the late 1960s and early 1970s, particularly the far-left 'Spartacus' movement with its campaign 'Öffnet die Heime' ('Open children's homes') performed activist and media-effective actions to point to cruelties in children's homes. This strategy was quite effective and led to the closing of the most violent institutions in the second half of the 1970s, accompanied by a strategic plan to reorganise the Austrian youth welfare system.

[8] The history and growing impact on the field of the Austrian independent living movement has only recently been the subject of an oral history project (Schönwiese et al, 2017). To learn more about the history of the independent living movement in Austria see: http://bidok.uibk.ac.at/projekte/behindertenbewegung/index.html

[9] Original quote: 'Ich leb dort vollbetreut. Das heißt, wenn ich sage, mich drückt ein Furz, dann rennen gleich alle her' (K7, in Kremsner, 2017, 188).

[10] Original quote: 'Es geht mir scheiße, es geht mir scheiße in dieser Hurens-Arsch-WG. Du würdest nicht einmal deine Kinder hier herschicken. Weil ich wohn drin und weiß ganz genau, wie Kinder behandelt werden. Du würdest das deinem Kind nicht freiwillig antun.' (K2, in Kremsner, 2017, 188).

References

Austrian Parliament (2014) Parlamentskorrespondenz Nr. 1241 vom 17.12.2014 [Parliament correspondence no. 1241 of 17 December 2014]. Available at: https://www.parlament.gv.at/PAKT/PR/JAHR_2014/PK1241/

Berger, E. (1996): 'Die psychiatrische Betreuung (geistig) behinderter Menschen' ['The psychiatric care of intellectually disabled persons'] in M. Moritz and E. Neck-Schaukowitsch (eds) *Beiträge zur Theorie und Praxis sozialer Dienste*, Vienna: Festschrift Wr. Sozialdienste, pp 85–91.

Biewer, G. (2009) *Grundlagen der Heilpädagogik und Inklusiven Pädagogik*, Bad Heilbrunn: Verlag Julius Klinkhardt.

Binding, K. and Hoche, A. (1920) *Die Freigabe der Vernichtung lebensunwerten Lebens: ihr Maß und ihre Form*, Leipzig: Meiner Verlag.

Buchner, T. (2009) 'Deinstitutionalisation and community living for people with intellectual disabilities in Austria: history, policies, implementation and research', *Tizard Learning Disability Review,* 14(1): 4-13.

Buchner, T. (2018) 'Biographische Erzählungen zu Persönlicher Assistenz: Kämpfe um Zugang, Ermöglichungen von Selbstbestimmung und ermächtigende Selbstdeutungen' ['Biographical narratives about Personal Assistance: fighting for access, facilitating self-determination and empowering self-constructions'], *SWS-Rundschau,* 52(2): 2-23.

Czech, H. (2002) 'Forschen ohne Skrupel. Die wissenschaftliche Verwertung von Opfern der NS-Fürsorge in Wien' ['Research without scruples: the scientific exploitation of victims of Nazi care in Vienna'] in E. Gabriel and W. Neugebauer (eds) *Von der Zwangssterilisierung zur Ermordung. Zur Geschichte der NS-Euthanasie in Wien,* Vienna: Böhlau, pp 143–63.

Czech, H. (2014) 'Der Spiegelgrund-Komplex. Kinderheilkunde, Heilpädagogik, Psychiatrie und Jugendfürsorge im Nationalsozialismus' ['The Spiegelgrund complex: paediatrics, curative education, psychiatry and youth welfare in National Socialism'] in M. Ralser and R. Sieder (eds) *Die Kinder des Staates/Children of the State,* Innsbruck: StudienVerlag, pp 194–219.

Droste, T. (1999) *Die Historie der Geistigbehindertenversorgung unter dem Einfluß der Psychiatrie seit dem 19.Jahrhundert. Eine kritische Analyse neuerer Entpsychiatrisierungsprogramme und geistigbehindertenpädagogischer Reformkonzepte* [*The history of mental handicap care under the influence of psychiatry since the 19th century: A critical analysis of de-psychiatrisation programmes and pedagogical reform concepts*], Münster, Hamburg & London: LIT-Verlag.

Forster, R. and Pelikan, M. (1978) *Patientenversorgung und Personalhandeln im Kontext einer psychiatrischen Sonderanstalt* [*Patient care and personnel acting in the context of a special psychiatric institution*], Vienna: IHS.

Häßler, G. and Häßler, F. (2005) *Geistig Behinderte im Spiegel der Zeit. Vom Narrenhäusl zur Gemeindepsychiatrie* [*Intellectually disabled people in the mirror of time: From the Fools' House to community psychiatry*], Stuttgart & New York: Thieme.

Heiss, G. (2015) *Endbericht für den Jubiläumsfonds der Österreichischen Nationalbank zum Forschungsprojekt „Die Malariatherapie und weitere diagnosekorrelierte Therapien: ihre Anwendung an der Wiener Universitätsklinik für Psychiatrie und Neurologie in den 1950er und 1960er Jahren und ihre Diskussion in der zeitgenössischen Forschung* [*Final report for the Jubilee Fund of the Austrian National Bank on the research project 'Malaria therapy and other diagnosis-related therapies: their application at the Viennese University Hospital of Psychiatry and Neurology in the 1950s and 1960s and their discussion in contemporary research'*], Not for publication. Personal copy – disclosed to third parties. Written consent to cite the study given by the author.

JG SPÖ NÖ (Junge Generation SPÖ Niederösterreich) (1980) *Protokoll über die Behindertenenquete 1978 der Jungen Generation in der SPÖ Niederösterreich am 25. November 1978 in Brunn am Gebirge* [*Protocol on the 1978 Disability Enquete of the Young Generation in the SPÖ Lower Austria on 25 November 1978 in Brunn am Gebirge*], Vienna: JG SPÖ NÖ.

Kosemund, A. (2005) *Spurensuche Irma. Berichte und Dokumente zur Geschichte der »Euthanasie-Morde« an Pfleglingen aus den Alsterdorfer Anstalten* [*Tracing Irma: Reports and documents on the history of the 'Euthanasia Murders' of inmates from the Alsterdorf region institutions*], Hamburg: Vereinigung der Verfolgten des Naziregimes -Bund der Antifaschistinnen und Antifaschisten (VVN-BdA).

Kremsner, G. (2017) *Vom Einschluss der Ausgeschlossenen zum Ausschluss der Eingeschlossenen. Biographische Erfahrungen von so genannten Menschen mit Lernschwierigkeiten* [*From confining the excluded to excluding the confined: Biographical experiences of so-called people with learning disabilities*], Bad Heilbrunn: Verlag Julius Klinkhardt.

Ledebur, S. (2015) *Das Wissen der Anstaltspsychiatrie in der Moderne. Zur Geschichte der Heil- und Pflegeanstalten Am Steinhof Wien* [*The knowledge of institutional psychiatry in modernity: On the history of the sanatoriums and nursing homes 'Am Steinhof' Vienna*], Vienna: Böhlau-Verlag.

Malina, P. (2007) 'Erziehungs-Terror: Politische und gesellschaftliche Voraussetzungen von Kindsein im Nationalsozialismus' ['Educational terror: political and social prerequisites for being a child during National Socialism'] in E. Berger (ed) *Verfolgte Kindheit. Kinder und Jugendliche als Opfer der NS-Sozialverwaltung*, Vienna: Böhlau, pp 91–106.

Mattner, D. (2000) *Behinderte Menschen in der Gesellschaft. Zwischen Ausgrenzung und Integration* [*Disabled people in society: Between exclusion and integration*], Stuttgart, Berlin and Cologne: Kohlhammer.

Mayrhofer, H., Wolfgruber, G., Geiger, K., Hammerschick, W. and Reidinger, V. (2017) (eds) *Kinder und Jugendliche mit Behinderungen in der Wiener Psychiatrie von 1945 bis 1989. Stationäre Unterbringung am Steinhof und Rosenhügel* [*Children and adolescents with disabilities in Viennese psychiatry from 1945 to 1989: Inpatient accommodation at Steinhof and Rosenhügel*], Vienna: LIT-Verlag.

Monitoringausschuss (2017) *Stellungnahme De-Institutionalisierung* [*Statement on deinstitutionalisation*]. Available at: https://monitoringausschuss.at/download/ma_sn_deinstitutionalisierung_final-pdf-2/

Plangger, S. and Schönwiese, V. (2010) 'Behindertenhilfe – Hilfe für behinderte Menschen? Geschichte und Entwicklungsphasen der Behindertenhilfe in Tirol' ['Care services – help for disabled people? History and development of care services for disabled persons in Tyrol'] in H. Schreiber (ed) *Im Namen der Ordnung. Heimerziehung in Tirol*, Innsbruck: StudienVerlag, pp 317–46.

Ralser, M. (2014) 'Psychiatrisierte Kindheit – Expansive Kulturen der Krankheit. Machtvolle Allianzen zwischen Psychiatrie und Fürsorgeerziehung' ['Psychiatricised childhood – expansive cultures of the disease: powerful alliances between psychiatry and child welfare education'] in M. Ralser and R. Sieder (eds) *Die Kinder des Staates/ Children of the State*, Innsbruck: StudienVerlag Innsbruck: Studien Verlag, pp 128–55.

Reichsgesetzblatt (1939) *Verordnung über die Einführung des Gesetzes zur Verhütung erbkranken Nachwuchses und des Gesetzes zum Schutze der Erbgesundheit des deutschen Volkes in der Ostmark vom 14. November 1939* [*Ordinance on the introduction of the law for the prevention of offspring with hereditary illness and the law to protect the hereditary health of the German people in the Ostmark, 14 November 1939*].

Schmidt, R. (1993) *Die Paläste der Irren. Kritische Betrachtungen zur Lebenssituation geistig behinderter Menschen in Österreich* [*Palaces of the lunatics: Critical reflections on the life situation of intellectually disabled people in Austria*], Vienna: WUV-Universitätsverlag.

Schönwiese, V. (2012) 'Individualisierende Eugenik – Zur Praxis von Andreas Rett' ['Individualising eugenics: Andreas Rett's practice'] in BIZEPS (ed) *Wertes unwertes Leben*, Vienna: BIZEPS, pp 69–82.

Schönwiese, V. (2013) *Thesen zur UN-Konvention über die Rechte von Menschen mit Behinderungen und die Perspektive der De-Institutionalisierung* [*Thesis on the UN Convention on the Rights of Persons with Disabilities and the perspective of deinstitutionalisation*]. Available at: http://bidok. uibk.ac.at/library/schoenwiese-thesen.html

Schönwiese, V., Plangger, S., Kremsner, G., Emberger, B. and Riegler, C. (2017) *Einleitungstext zum Archiv zur Geschichte der Behindertenbewegung – SELBSTBESTIMMT LEBEN BEWEGUNG in Österreich von 1945 bis 2008* [*Introduction to the archive on the history of the Disabled People's Movement in Austria from 1945 to 2008*]. Available at: http://bidok.uibk.ac.at/projekte/behindertenbewegung/geschichte.html.

Sieder, R. (2014) 'Das Dispositiv der Fürsorgeerziehung in Wien' ['The dispositive of welfare education in Vienna'] in M. Ralser and R. Sieder (eds) *Die Kinder des Staates/Children of the State*, Innsbruck: StudienVerlag, pp 156–93.

SLIÖ (2014) *SLIÖ-Positionspapier zu Biopolitik* [*SLIÖ Position Paper on Biopolitics*]. Available at: https://cdn.website-editor.net/d23c59d4124842da9c555afcbfca6c43/files/uploaded/2014%2520SLI%25C3%2596%2520Positionspapier%2520zur%2520Bio-Politik.pdf

Strachota, A. (2002) *Heilpädagogik und Medizin. Eine Beziehungsgeschichte* [*Special needs education and medicine: A relationship (hi)story*], Vienna: Literas Universitätsverlag.

Weiss, H. (1978) 'Geschichte der Psychiatrie in Österreich' ['History of psychiatry in Austria'], *Österreichische Zeitschrift für Soziologie*, 3(2), 41–57.

Westermann, G. and Buchner, T. (2008) 'Erfahrungsbericht. Die Lebensgeschichte von Gerhard Westermann' ['The life story of Gerhard Westermann'] in E. Boehlke (ed) *Individuelle Biografieforschung als Entwicklungschance für Menschen mit Intelligenzminderung*, Berlin: Edition GIB, pp 120–144 .

Zemp, A. and Pircher, E. (1996) *Weil das alles weh tut mit Gewalt. Sexuelle Ausbeutung von Mädchen und Frauen mit Behinderung* [*Because it all hurts with violence: Sexual exploitation of girls and women with disabilities*], Vienna: Bundesministerin für Frauenangelegenheiten und Verbraucherschutz.

THREE

Time of paradoxes: what the twentieth century was like for people with intellectual disabilities living in Czechoslovakia/Czech Republic

Monika Mužáková and Iva Strnadová

Introduction

The twentieth century was marked by a number of political and policy shifts that impacted the lives of people with intellectual disabilities and their families. Some were worldwide (eg two World Wars), while others (eg the onset and fall of totalitarianism) were specific to the Czech Republic, but all influenced perceptions of and attitudes towards people with intellectual disabilities.

The authors use the terminology in use at the time, to keep the chapter historically accurate. Readers will encounter outdated terms: 'feeble-minded', 'idiots', 'mentally handicapped'. As Sinason commented, it is 'doing a grave disservice to past pioneers to point contemptuously to their chosen terms. Within another five years, the process of euphemism will already be affecting the brave new words' (Sinason, 2010, 35).

Antecedents: pre-twentieth century

Approximately three hundred and fifty years ago, Czech scholar Comenius (1592–1670) said that no human being is beyond the power of education. Little did he know how many people would declassify this thought, and for how many people it would become hope and inspiration. Comenius' belief that it was not possible to find a person of such mental incapacity for whom education would not bring any improvement at all was, however, long to be fulfilled. It wasn't until the nineteenth century, when the first specialised institutions were built, that society began to seek a humanly reasonable relationship towards people with intellectual disabilities. Although these institutions were segregated, education was introduced to assist people in developing self-care and work habits.

The first institution in the Austro-Hungarian Empire, the 'Institution of Idiots', was founded by physician and educator Karel Slavoj Amerling (1807–84) in 1871. Amerling combined medical and educational interventions (Herfort, 1932). He created an education system graded according to the level of intellectual disability, rather than age. He built on students' prior knowledge in teaching. The curriculum included craft instruction. The goal was to return the child to family care, or to support him/her to be successful in adulthood by acquiring manual work skills. Amerling introduced music therapy (Černá et al, 2008), and prohibited physical punishment.

The possibilities of education for the feeble-minded (1900–18)

Around 1900, the idea of compulsory education for children with mild intellectual disabilities within the existing school system arose. Teachers, physicians, social workers and officials sought a way to help these children to use their knowledge and skills.

The first auxiliary class for feeble-minded students was opened in Prague in 1896 (Titzl, 2016). The name 'auxiliary' was deduced from the word 'to help'. The aim was the optimal reduction of the curriculum and the use of special teaching methods. Emphasis was put on the professional training of teachers who taught these children. The greatest progress was made in this area by František Čáda (1865–1918), philosopher and college educator. He promoted the idea of social consensus and interdisciplinary cooperation in the newly formed system of education for feeble-minded children. He supported the organisation of three Czech Congresses on care for the feeble-minded and schooling for the feeble-minded in 1909, 1911 and 1913. Čáda believed that the state, not charity, should take responsibility for these citizens (Congress Committee, 1909). He advocated that persons with intellectual disabilities should receive support for transition from special schools to apprenticeships or supported jobs, where they could work according to their ability. Čáda argued that people with intellectual disabilities should receive enough support to be able to contribute to and be part of society, an idea not out of place in the twenty-first century.

Professor Karel Herfort (1871–1940), the founder of Czech child psychiatry, pioneered work with people who were severely mentally handicapped. He viewed the care of the 'mentally handicapped' as a moral commitment, a gift and a challenge. He was Amerling's successor as head of the Institution of Idiots, and elevated it to a world-class level, drawing on his wide foreign experience. He introduced classes for severely disabled students, corrective physical training and needlework. He designed teaching aids and considered manual activity and play the most effective way of educating these students. He sought the possibility of speech correction and targeted the development of fine and gross motor skills. He pointed out the necessity of educative and loving stimulation of even the most severely disabled students (Herfort, 1932).

He published widely in Czech, German, and French, emphasising the importance of familiarising trainee doctors with the cognitive development of individuals with intellectual disabilities, and arguing for the need to have the best teachers for these students. Unfortunately, these ideals have even now not been completely fulfilled.

This quest for improved teaching methods and ways of communication clashed with eugenic campaigns. Feeble-mindedness was seen through the prism of unproductiveness of the 'unfit', who endanger the 'fit' and 'racially pure'.

> Intelligence was abstracted to one single trait which was placed in the brain and then quantified into one single number and these numbers were then used to rank people according to their value. All this happened repeatedly in order to conclude that suppressed and disadvantaged groups of people (races, classes, genders) are born as inferior and therefore they deserve their inferior position. (Gould, 1997, 50)

Eugenicists blamed the feeble-minded for a worsening economic situation, putting prosperity at stake. Eugenics sparked contemplation in the Czech lands about whether the 'inferior', among whom feeble-minded persons were categorised, had the right to belong in our world. Earlier attempts to 'eliminate the sickness rate and abnormality by regulating marriage' (Růžička, 1923, 572) and to 'bring back normal constitution to people and reproduce it' (Růžička, 1923, 572) were facing the belief that '… society definitely isn't supposed to take care of preserving the second-class descendants, but to take care of reproducing socially valuable progeny' (Veselá, 1937, 38). Being sympathetic to the feeble-minded was a luxury, incompatible with the vision of a just society, endangering the security of full-value citizens and the success of the state.

Karel Herfort made people appreciate unique capabilities in disabled people and he did so at a time when sterilisation was a widely canvassed option. Herfort studied the heredity of feeble-mindedness. He established in Ernestinum (1913) a 'private eugenic station', a register of the feeble-minded, which also created their family trees. Herfort developed questionnaires to be completed by the parents of his students to find out if the genes of feeble-mindedness were present in the family. He was well aware that his research had its limits, and sounded a note of caution for concluding on the provenance of feeble-mindedness:

> Genetic burden can be considered the real cause of feeble-mindedness only if it led to feeble-mindedness in all cases. Does the same cause in our cases have the same consequences as in physics and chemistry? We know that it doesn't. (Herfort, 1915, quoted in Herfort, 1932, 172)

Herfort showed that families with feeble-minded children also had children who were not feeble-minded, and who were frequently gifted. In his view, no scientific theory regarding people with disability should serve as a justification for their segregation. Herfort recognised that rationality and progress are not enough to understand another human being. Prominent eugenicist Vladislav Růžička asked: 'Wouldn't it be obvious to wonder if the whole eugenic effort isn't only a manifestation of futile desire to achieve ideals?' (1923, 571). This doubt may have contributed to the fact that the Czech eugenic movement failed to instigate repressive interventions of an eliminatory nature. At a time when eugenic visions and forced sterilisations were happening in other parts of Europe and America, Czech special education achieved one of its peaks.

Auxiliary schools (1918–48)

Czechoslovakia came into existence in 1918. The new republic began to build a primary school system. The term 'auxiliary schooling' was used from 1918 for the whole system of special schools for students with visual, hearing, physical and intellectual impairments.

Josef Zeman (1867–1961), a talented and devoted teacher, helped to create new institutions for handicapped children. Together with Karel Herfort, he is considered the greatest authority in Czechoslovak special education between the wars. Zeman believed that a quality network of schools for the severely handicapped would benefit all of those 'pushed aside' (Zeman, 1909). He showed extraordinary organisational abilities when appointed as an inspector of the auxiliary school system at the Ministry of Education and National Education in 1919. Places increased from 293 in 29 classes in 1920 to 1,714 in 111 classes in 1938 (Titzl, 2016).

Zeman influenced the political climate and public opinion to become more favourable to handicapped children. His *Curricula and Educational Plans for Auxiliary Schools* received support in 1928, and Law 86 on auxiliary schools (classes) was passed in 1929.

Zeman's attempts to promote secondary schools for mentally handicapped students were based on the assumption that these children need work and life skills so that as adults they can become independent and make a living. Zeman appreciated that unemployment brought about not only a social gap, but also the stigma of exclusion (Zeman, 1939). He succeeded in establishing higher education for teachers at auxiliary schools and lectured in the newly opened courses. He focused on raising awareness among mainstream elementary school teachers, since many believed that auxiliary school teachers knew less because they taught children who knew less.

In 1924 Zeman and Herfort founded the journal, *Deviant Youth*, which focused on gaining new scientific knowledge to improve the care of handicapped children. Its objective was to spark an interest in leading Czech scientists in conducting research in this field.

In 1930 Zeman wrote:

> Times are changing and culture with it. Opinions on the child are changing, pedagogical science is developing in recent years, especially pedopathology. Until recently, child care used to be of a rather philanthropic and social nature, however, nowadays it is eminently a question of education. (p 5)

Zeman's thinking can be linked to the intention of other representatives of special education in Czechoslovakia to help children through the introduction of modern teaching methods. Auxiliary schools for students with intellectual disabilities thus achieved a high level of quality in Czechoslovakia, compared with the most progressive European countries.

This changed dramatically during the Second World War and occupation of Czechoslovakia from 1938 to 1945. It proved easy to use the prevailing hatred towards people who were different and apply it to those with intellectual disabilities. People with intellectual disabilities and mental illness became defenceless victims of the most atrocious ideology: Nazi euthanasia. They were targeted and liquidated during 'operation T4' in the so-called Protectorate of Bohemia and Moravia. Most of the approximately 1,100 patients murdered between December 1940 and July 1941 came from general medical and nursing institutions in Bohemia and Moravia. Between 1942 and 1945, more than 600 patients of Jewish origin, including children with severe intellectual disabilities or mental illness, were tortured to death or murdered (Šimůnek et al, 2009).

Special education and institutions during totalitarianism (1948–1989)

The totalitarian regime which came into being after the Second World War sought to control all areas of everyday life.

> The peak achievement of communist education should have been ... a more or less perfect person who isn't attached to his/her private possessions and who can live in harmony with others. (Hábl and Janiš, 2010, 108)

Soon after the communist regime came into power, Law No. 95/1948 on the Basic Regulation of the Unified School System was adopted. Schools for students with mild intellectual disabilities became a part of the unified school system, which can be seen as a very positive outcome. The same applied to schools for students with physical and sensory impairments. The number of students with mild intellectual disabilities in special schools grew during the communist era: from 7,843 in 1949 to 58,889 in 1989 (Titzl, 2016). These schools had excellent textbooks, and the curriculum was revised periodically. Emphasis was put on teaching Czech to develop speech and thinking. In addition, schools offered craft lessons to develop working skills and manual dexterity (Titzl, 2016). Compulsory school attendance was eight or nine years, and then students left for apprenticeships. Their employability was subsequently good, and because there was high equalisation of salaries in communist Czechoslovakia, people with mild intellectual disabilities did not end up on the edge of society.

Nevertheless, this regime, which built its existence on the ideology of equality, created two categories of people: the 'educable' and the 'uneducable'. Those who were unable to meet the demands of a special school were deprived of the opportunity to learn. Thus, there were thousands of people with severe levels of intellectual disabilities who had no support at all. The regime tried to segregate them into specialised institutions. The state assumed that in institutions all their needs can be fulfilled, and at the same time, by placing these people behind walls, the state would solve the question of a 'new man', not burdened by the past, healthy and efficient. Despite this, throughout the communist era, most people with severe levels of intellectual disabilities lived with their families, because there were too few places in institutions (Mužáková, 2016).

There was little to no interest in the day-to-day lives of people with more severe forms of intellectual disabilities. The politics of exclusivity in communist Czechoslovakia was not reflected in direct care provided by the state (Marková and Středová, 1987), but rather in attempts to make them 'invisible'. As one father commented: "These people were hidden somewhere because communists didn't want to admit that they had handicapped children. You knew where the institutions were located … in hidden places" (Mr Horčík, in Mužáková, 2016, 30). Mainstream society was not informed about people with severe levels of intellectual disabilities and their way of living, either with their families or in institutional care, and was deprived of the possibility to respect or understand them as fellow human beings.

There was some improvement in the early 1960s. Thanks to Miloš Sovák (1905–89), the first kindergarten for children with intellectual disabilities opened in Prague in 1960. In the same year the term 'auxiliary school' re-appeared, but in a different context. Schools for students with moderate levels of intellectual disabilities were called auxiliary schools, and schools for students with other types of disabilities were called special schools. According to Law 186/1960, students with moderate intellectual disabilities could receive education in auxiliary schools for two years, and afterwards went to a special school or were exempt from compulsory education. The law was a result of lobbying by parents. The establishment of auxiliary schools was progress, but only for some; children who could not be educated in auxiliary schools were still labelled 'uneducable'.

Deeds to respect (1968–89)

Despite the consolidation of dictatorship in Czechoslovakia, some individual attempts to fight injustice stand out. Parents of children with severe intellectual disabilities, whose main goal was to lessen the public stigmatisation and social inequality of their offspring, initiated incredible reforms. It wasn't easy to fight in the shadow of oppression, social discrimination and the demands of everyday care. It wasn't easy to fight against the humiliation of their own children (Mužáková, 2016).

However, some parents found courage to speak out. These parents believed that despite their children's seeming limitations, they also needed human contact, mutuality and understanding.

Božena Gürtlerová (1915–2017), a mother of a daughter with Down's Syndrome, linked her fate with those of similar families to establish a volunteer humanitarian association in Czechoslovakia. After ten years of dealing with authorities, who initially considered her proposals that parents of mentally handicapped children should have their own organisation undoable, the Association for Help to the Mentally Handicapped in the Czech Republic (SPMP) came into existence in September 1969. The Association presented proposals for institutions for adolescents and adults, run on a weekly basis. People would stay there during the week and return to their families for weekends and holidays (Titzl, 2005).

Achievements in the field of counselling enabled families with mentally disabled children to have more frequent contact with their offspring placed in a permanent social care institution. This allowed the Association to focus on a dialogue with specialists to ensure better medical care, rehabilitation and education.

Thanks to these efforts, the Association also succeeded in reforming existing institutions, achieved some progress in the education of children with more severe disabilities, and supported leisure activities. They organised dance and swimming lessons, rehabilitation stays, trips, and sporting events for families and their children. They contributed to attendance at auxiliary school being extended to eight years in 1978.

To conclude, the totalitarian social order gave people the idea that it would solve all human justice issues. However, the original intended collective responsibility soon turned into collective irresponsibility, which affected the most vulnerable citizens.

Following the Velvet Revolution (1989–2000)

The changes that occurred after the so-called Velvet Revolution in 1989 were based on developments during communism: 'no epoch develops its teachings on its own, but carries on with (intentionally or unknowingly, favourably or disapprovingly) the thoughts of the previous era' (Rádl, 2006, vol I, 57).

In 1991, a Government Committee for Persons with Disability was established, which developed a National Plan of Actions for Persons with Disability in 1992. Although not legally binding, changes suggested by this National Plan were slowly introduced and implemented. By 1993, 'the Czech Republic was recognized as being among the countries with the most advanced national concept of support for citizens with disability' (Vann and Šiška, 2006, 430).

Following the country's newly gained freedom in November 1989, there was a gradual transformation of institutional care. Yet, according to estimates by Inclusion Europe and The Association for Help to the Mentally Handicapped in the Czech Republic, approximately 15,000 people with intellectual disabilities remained institutionalised in approximately 143 institutions in 1998 (Inclusion Europe and SPMP, 2002; Vann and Šiška 2006). Supported employment was gradually established, and larger institutions reformed (Nelb Sinecká, 2013). While deinstitutionalisation began after 1989, there was in 2018 still a long road ahead before the elimination of all institutions in the Czech Republic (Vann and Šiška, 2006).

Another shift in post-communist times was a change in social care provision. The state de-monopolised its role in the provision of social care in 1990, which led to rapid growth in non-governmental organisations and new services, focusing on 'day services, small-scale residential accommodation, and vocational training programs' (Vann and Šiška, 2006, 433).

The education of people with intellectual disabilities was influenced by international trends. After the fall of communism (1989–2000), efforts were made to correct previous injustices by introducing compulsory education for all children. However, it was not until 2004 that a law was passed, stating that all children without exception have the right to be educated. As a result, special schools for students with severe and profound intellectual disabilities were established. Furthermore, the first efforts to introduce integration in mainstream schools began, and opportunities for lifelong education for adults with intellectual disabilities started to appear.

Life story: Anthony

What was the impact of recent Czech history on the everyday lives of people with intellectual disabilities, their parents and loved ones? Through an interview with the mother of a child with intellectual disabilities in 2015, the authors sought to understand what life was like for a mentally handicapped child and his family in communist Czechoslovakia.

Anthony was born in 1981 in a large industrial town in northern Bohemia. He was the second child. His birth was without complications, but Anthony's development, in comparison to that of his older and younger brothers, made his mother aware of his delayed psychomotor development, and led to her seeking help from a psychologist. She remembered this as a time of uncertainty. She gained financial support from the state and was informed by a psychiatrist that Anthony had a profound and permanent cognitive impairment without any possibility of improvement. Examination at a neurological clinic in Prague confirmed a hypotonic form of cerebral palsy. Anthony was enrolled in a local special kindergarten, where he was happy. At home, he was restless and hyperactive. His mother was left mostly alone in caring for him, as his father went to work and grandparents lived at a distance. People expected her to manage, as she was a special educator. She realised that responsibility for all decisions related to Anthony would be hers. She did not receive any advice or assistance, only the recommendation to place Anthony in an institution.

She taught in a special school where most of the children were from Roma families. She told us Anthony could not be accepted there, as his disability was too severe. As a result, he was exempt from school attendance. His parents placed Anthony in an institution on a weekly basis in a nearby town. However, Anthony's behaviour became less manageable at home during weekends, the parents were completely exhausted, and they also feared for the healthy development of Anthony's siblings, although they enjoyed playing and talking with their brother. When Anthony was nine, his parents made a difficult decision – to place him into a year-round institution for boys. She recalled:

> "... it was a terrible moment, terrible, I did not experience anything worse, and I do not think I will ever experience anything this terrible again. He was nine years old, and it was an institution all the way up in the outpost in the north of the republic, and we just left him in such place. [Our son] thought he was going for a trip, we bought him a pair of shoes on the way, and we left him there and went home. ... it was a really ghastly thing, and then I had to drive [our car] back so that I could hold on to the wheel, otherwise I would go crazy about what we did... and then such desperation, a terrible feeling of emptiness and grievous guilt, even if it was clear that there was no other solution. ... We visited him regularly, but it was awful ... it was just a torture for him, as there was just one visiting Sunday per month. It was also terribly far... Sometimes we took him home for a weekend but that did not make us happy, the first evening was good, he was back with us but then time fled terribly fast, and we brought him back to that gruesome house, it was really hard."

Parents and siblings regularly visited Anthony. Their belief in God was their support; however, Anthony could not practise his faith in the institution.

The Velvet Revolution in 1989 and fall of the communist regime brought new hope. The parents looked for a place where their son would be happy. In 1995, when Anthony was 14, his family moved to Prague, and Anthony was placed in a home run by a charity.

> "This home was a community of beautiful people. It was shortly after the revolution, they played the guitar, sang songs, and had so much respect for the people [with severe and profound disabilities]. Finally, we managed, this is how I always imagined it. Anthony was still displaying challenging behaviours … how many times did it come to me that he seemed to have completely calmed down. … Every time I come there, and he's always shaved, dressed, laughing, and every time when I bring him back there and he's looking forward to it, I just really feel a deep gratitude. … Everything for us here in Prague was all new and thanks to this we felt that we belonged somewhere. We belong to a beautiful society. …"

At the time of the interview, in 2015, Anthony still lived in this home where he has friends and feels useful. He goes home every weekend, and his siblings keep in contact with him, and if necessary, are ready to help Anthony's mother, who continues to work as a special educator and is convinced that through her own experience she can better understand the concerns of parents of the children she teaches. She has great satisfaction that her son is doing well in the home, and thanks to this she can continue in her employment. The most valuable thing for her is her gratitude to the staff at Anthony's home who understand and help her son. The family is convinced that this small community home is the best place for Anthony.

References

Černá, M., Strnadová, I., Šiška, J., Titzl, B. and Kainová, T. (2008) *Česká psychopedie (Czech psychopedy: Special education of people with intellectual disabilities)*, Prague: Karolinum.

Congress Committee (eds) (1909) *Prvý český sjezd pro péči o slabomyslné a školství pomocné (The first Czech congress on care for the feeble-minded and for auxiliary schooling)*, Prague: Nákladem sjezdového výboru.

Gould, J.S. (1997) *Jak neměřit člověka (How not to measure a man)*, Prague: Nakladatelství Lidové noviny.

Hábl, J. and Janiš, K. ml (2010) *Přehled dějin pedagogiky (Overview of the history of education)*, Hradec Králové: Gaudeamus.

Herfort, K. (1932) 'Eugenický význam slabomyslnsoti a prvé výsledky prací v tomto směrů vykonaných eugenickou stanicí při Ernestinu 1915' ('The eugenic meaning of the feeble-mindedness and the first results of the work carried out in this area by the eugenic station by Ernestinum 1915'), in J. Zeman (ed) *Soubor prací univ. Prof. MUDR. Karla Herforta (Collection of works of university professor MUDR. Karel Herfort)*, Prague: Spolek pro péči o slabomyslné, pp 177–99.

Inclusion Europe (The European Association of Societies of Persons with Intellectual Disability and their Families) and SPMP (The Association for Help to the Mentally Handicapped in the Czech Republic) (2002) in J. Šiška, *Human rights of persons with intellectual disability. Country report: Czech Republic*, Brussels: Inclusion Europe.

Marková, Z. and Středová, L. (1987) *Mentálně postižené dítě v rodině (Mentally handicapped child in a family)*, Prague: Státní pedagogické nakladatelství.

Mužáková, M. (2016) *Byly to naše děti. O fenoménu lásky a sounáležitosti s rodiči a jejich dětmi s mentálním postižením v každodennosti totality (They were our children: The phenomenon of love and belonging, and parents and their children with intellectual disabilities in the everydayness of totalitarianism)*, Prague: Charles University, Faculty of Education.

Nelb Sinecká, J. (2013) 'Nahlédnutí za zeď: Deinstitutionalizace lidí s autismem za komunismu a po roce 1989 v narativech rodičů' ('Looking over the wall: deinstitutionalization of people with autism during communism and after 1989 in parental narratives'), *Sociální práce*, 1, 37–48.

Rádl, E. (2006) *Dějiny biologických teorií novověku (History of biological theories of modern times)*, vols I and II, Prague: Academia.

Růžička, V. (1923) *Biologické základy eugeniky (Biological origins of eugenics)*, Prague: Fr. Borový.

Šimůnek, M., Böhm, B., Eigeisberger, P., Fedorovič, T., Schulze, D., Schwanninger, F. and Zeman, P. (2009) *Nehodné žití: nacistická 'eutanázie' v říšské župě Sudety a protektorátu Čechy a Morava, 1939–1945 (Unworthy living: Nazi 'euthanasia' in the Sudetenland and Protectorate of Bohemia and Moravia, 1939–1945)*, Katalog. Verein Schloss Hartheim.

Sinason, V. (2010) *Mental handicap and the human condition: An analytic approach to intellectual disability* (revised edn), London: Free Association Books.

Titzl, B. (2005) 'Politika totalitního (totalitárního) režimu vůči zdravotně postiženým občanům' ('Totalitarian (totalitarian) policy towards disabled citizens'), in H. Nosková et al (eds), *K problémům menšin v Československu v letech 1945–1989. Sborník studií (Proceedings of studies)*, Prague: Ústav pro soudobé dějiny AV ČR, pp 21–61.

Titzl, B. (2016) 'Naučit nebo inkludovat?' ('To teach or to include?'), *Speciální pedagogika (Special Education)*, 3, 261–93.

Vann, B.H. and Šiška, J. (2006) 'From "cage beds" to inclusion: the long road for individuals with ID in the Czech Republic', *Disability & Society*, 21, 425–39. doi: 10.1080/09687590600785811

Veselá, J. (1938) *Sterilizace: problém populační, sociální a kriminální politik (Sterilisation: A problem of population, social and criminal policy)*, Prague: Mazáč.

Zeman, J. (1930) *Svět nevidomých (The world of the blind)*, Prague: Dědictví Komenského.

Zeman, J. (1939) *Dějiny péče o slabomyslné (The history of care for the feeble-minded)*, Prague: Spolek pro péči o slabomyslné.

FOUR

Intellectual disability in twentieth-century Ghana

Jane Abraham and Auberon Jaleel Odoom

Ghana, a country in West Africa with a current population of just under 30 million, was a British colony until 1957 (previously called the Gold Coast), when it became the first colony in sub-Saharan Africa to regain its independence.

Prior to independence, Britain, as the colonial power, extracted natural resources – gold, diamonds, timber and cocoa. Britain built railways and transport systems to assist resource extraction. A few Western–style hospitals and schools were built, with the education system geared to training a Ghanaian elite to run the country on Britain's behalf, at least initially. Many schools were modelled on British boarding schools and run by missionaries and educators from Britain and other European countries. However, day-to-day life for the majority of Ghanaians – including those with disabilities – was little touched by the colonisers, being determined rather by local tradition, chiefs and clan elders. In the latter part of the twentieth century, increasing urbanisation and technological development began to drive more significant changes in lifestyle and attitudes, particularly in urban areas.

Recognition of intellectual disability and lack of visible presence of people with intellectual disability in Ghana

Throughout the twentieth century, there seems to have been little visible presence of persons with intellectual disability. This was in part because persons with mild disabilities tended to be relatively well integrated in their village/clan/family group in Ghana, especially in rural areas where subsistence agriculture was (and remains) dominant, and literacy was relatively unimportant. On the other hand, persons with more profound impairments often did not survive infancy.

The development of educational provision during the twentieth century increased the visibility of some children with disabilities. At the time, it was assumed these children were unable to access mainstream education. Some special schools were started, the first being the Blind

School in Mampong, founded in 1945 by Basel Missionaries. The first special school for children with intellectual disabilities was Dzorwulu Special School in Accra, founded in 1970. But although intellectual disability was sometimes recognised, there were no systematic records kept. Indeed, there are still few statistics and little research on intellectual disabilities in Ghana, and no reliable figures on how many people there are. Within Ghana there was no standard definition, and a lack of recognised professionals able to monitor and assess people. This meant 'scientific testing and the medical models of disability tend to not be so prominent' (quote from an Inclusion Ghana information booklet). Even when people were informally labelled, the information was generally not officially recorded. A lack of resources and services meant there was little incentive for either the authorities, or people and their families, to use this label. Another reason for the lack of visibility was that the typically very negative view of disabilities in Ghanaian society meant many people, particularly with more profound disabilities, were kept hidden or neglected, or were actively killed. Infanticide of newborn children with intellectual disabilities still occurs, particularly in rural Ghana.

There was little institutionalisation either prior to or post Ghana's independence. A partial exception is the main psychiatric hospital in Accra, where some of the patients had an intellectual disability. The causes and treatment (if any) for both mental ill-health and intellectual disability were considered similar.

Inclusion and exclusion

Community attitudes can be gauged from some of the vocabulary used. Within major Ghanaian languages there are specific negative words, for example 'Asotowo' (meaning idiot in Ewe) and 'Buulu' (meaning stupid in Ga), that are used to refer to people with intellectual disabilities, demonstrating a lack of respect. Similarly, those with Down's Syndrome are labelled 'nsuoba' meaning spirit or water children in Twi. The various negative labels contribute to creating an excluded group (Agbenyega, 2003). The presence in some Ghanaian folk stories of creatures who are not quite human may also represent people with intellectual disabilities.

A child born with disabilities in a village would often be left to die in the bush or by the river. This was seen as allowing the child's spirit to return to the spirit realm, so it could be reborn in a 'proper' body in the future. It is notable that as a result of high infant and maternal mortality rates, even 'normal' newborn children in Ghana remained (and remain) unnamed and uncelebrated for the first few days of life, in case they died (seen as returning to the spirit world) in this period.

Whilst there were few residential institutions in Ghana where people might be segregated, it was common for people with more severe intellectual disabilities who survived the danger of infanticide to be excluded from full life within the community even when living in the family home, by being kept secluded or locked up, and typically unmentioned. On the other hand, those with milder impairments could be relatively well integrated.

Causes of disability

Underpinning the generally negative views of disabled people in Ghana was the widely held belief that everything had a spiritual cause. The continued centrality of faith and belief in spiritual causation means that to be accepted as valid by most Ghanaians, models of disability need to include a spiritual element that addresses both the causes of disability and how to respond to it (Hervie, 2013).

A disability was often believed to be due to a curse on the family, to be a consequence of a bargain by the family with evil spiritual forces, or to be a punishment for bad behaviour by parents or grandparents. Such explanations tended to reinforce stigmatisation and exclusion of both the person with intellectual disabilities and their family. Even where a person's disability was not viewed as the result of a curse, religious beliefs continued to influence how people were viewed by the public, their immediate families and themselves (Anthony, 2010). These attitudes and beliefs are still held by the majority in Ghana. The Ashanti people see disability as punishment from the gods and therefore tend to exclude people with disabilities from some or all of community life. However, decisions on specific cases typically depend on the elders of the community or family heads. For example, whether a child is hidden away or allowed to work, say on the family farm, will be determined by kinsfolk. A more positive example is that the Ga people of southern Ghana believe in reincarnation and sometimes view people with disabilities as reincarnations of the ancestors who have come back to give the community another chance to care for them and treat them well (Nukunya, 2003)

Negative beliefs about the causes of intellectual disability are also prevalent in Ghanaian churches, which are hugely influential. At the end of the twentieth century, 69% of Ghana's population self-reported as Christian (and a further 16% as Muslim). Many churches taught that illness, often including disabilities, is from the Devil, and should be expected to be healed by God. Church prayer camps in rural areas were popular. People with particular needs would go to these for extended periods of intense prayer. As reported in television documentaries (Al Jazeera, 2013; BBC, 2015), prayer camps are still sometimes places where children with intellectual disabilities are harshly treated albeit with the aim of achieving a 'cure'.

Religion in Ghana has often reinforced stigma, exclusion and maltreatment, although supportive faith communities have also been sources of acceptance and encouragement.

Human rights?

Following independence, Ghana's new Constitution embedded the rights of people with disabilities as 'citizens of Ghana'. Towards the end of the twentieth century, Article 29 of the 1992 Constitution guaranteed basic rights for people with disabilities and this was later supported by a legal framework, the Disability Law, Act 715 (2006). The implementation of these rights has been slow, and in the case of intellectual disability, often non-existent.

One reason is that much of Ghanaian society, including many law-makers, do not see disability rights law as applying to persons with intellectual disabilities (Baffoe, 2013). The starting point to have effective rights is society recognising that 'people with intellectual disabilities are human beings too' (personal communication, Maame Yaa, self-advocate, 2016).

Negative societal views remain obvious,[1] although this is now increasingly being challenged. The drive for change has been spearheaded by parents. Parent organisations, such as the Parent Association of Children with Intellectual Disability (PACID),[2] have been a mainstay of support and advocacy. They have also been crucial in educating and supporting parents themselves.

Historically, the lack of respect for persons with intellectual disability has been seen within the disability movement as well as wider society. Part of the momentum to start Inclusion Ghana and its member groups was the wish for persons with intellectual disabilities to become included as full members within disability umbrella groups at local and national levels.

Access to education

An important issue is how people were able to access, and were treated by, the education system. This is both a key indicator of how well inclusion is working, and strongly determinative of how views of people with disabilities might change over time, as school children grow into adults and become leaders in society.

Before and after independence in 1957, young people with mild to moderate disabilities were trained in trades like many of their non-disabled peers, and as noted above, the first special school for children with intellectual disability opened in 1970. In 1988 there were 17 special schools overseen by the Ministry of Education.

The 1990s marked early steps by the Ministry of Education, working with UNESCO (the United Nations Educational, Scientific and Cultural Organization), to develop an integrated education system. This principally focused on starting 'integrated schools' for children with intellectual disabilities, where a small number of 'special' classrooms were attached to regular schools. Children would be segregated in these 'special' classrooms. The aim was to give disabled and non-disabled children opportunities to interact socially on their shared school site. Even at the time, this approach was seen by some Ghanaian policy makers as an interim step towards inclusive schools (with children with intellectual disabilities mainstreamed in standard classrooms), and since 2003, inclusive education has been the emphasis of policy, at least for children with mild or moderate disabilities.

However, since schools tended to teach in traditional ways and had limited resources, with large classes, learning by rote and copying, inclusion, particularly of children with intellectual disabilities, was difficult. A former special education teacher lecturer told us how in the final years of the twentieth century when he was training teachers on how they could work with disabled children, other education lecturers actively promoted the inclusion of children with visual and hearing impairments, but advised their students that it was too difficult to integrate children with intellectual disabilities.

Another factor tending to limit educational opportunities has been that even parents with financial means may prefer to focus their resources for education on any children they have without disabilities, seeing it as a waste to spend money on educating a child with intellectual disabilities.

Vocational training and work

Once children had left the formal education system, there were some efforts to promote inclusion of people with disabilities in both training and employment. However, since 1992 only persons with severe disabilities have been referred to rehabilitation centres and offered training. There were 38 such centres (National Vocational Training Centres) throughout the country. All vocational training (except in the capital city) was focused on rural crafts such as basket-weaving, bead-making, shoe-making, and tie-and-dye. After completing the training programme, it was hoped people would be able to find work to support themselves, although this has often not happened.

As has been the case for many decades, Ghana has high unemployment. Employers were (and remain) reluctant to take on people with disabilities, particularly given that they have many applicants who have no disability to choose from. In addition, many employers felt that employment of persons with disabilities might bring bad luck to a company or to other workers, or that products made by them might somehow be contaminated. For example, bakery projects staffed by persons with intellectual disabilities in both Cape Coast and Accra had to stop selling their bread, as local market stallholders would not buy it due to concerns that customers might feel it would bring them bad luck, or even disability.

Family life and marriageability

In the twentieth century, another factor impacting on people's role and treatment was the economic contribution to parents and family expected from children as they grew up, and when they became adults. As in many other relatively poor countries, children's current and future economic contribution was often vital for parents and families, given that pensions were (and remain) generally inadequate or absent altogether. However, children with intellectual disabilities were usually viewed as a likely lifelong financial drain rather than as future contributors to family economic well-being. A lack of positive roles in the community (including a lack of employment opportunities) contributed to this concern for families.

Key potential roles within the community were to marry and to become a parent. Whether someone with intellectual disabilities was seen as a possible marriage partner has varied across time and location. For example, we were told of one woman who had married and had children. She was supported by her family. Both her children (a girl and a boy) also had an intellectual disability. When they became adults, the girl was sterilised. This decision was made by the wider family, who did not feel the girl would be capable of parenting adequately, and were not willing to provide the ongoing support that had been provided for the mother.

We now discuss two life stories of Ghanaian self-advocates, whose lives illustrate some of the points discussed above.

Maame Yaa's story: "We are human beings too"

Maame Yaa was born in 1990. She was born in a rural area but was brought up in Tema, an industrialising city and port near the capital, Accra. At the age of about 10, she was sent to live at Echoing Hills (a non-government organisation – NGO – on the outskirts of Accra which works with adults and children with disabilities and also provided a safe place for orphans). She gives some insight into the impact on her of positive family views of her, negative community views, access to education, dreams and aspirations.

Moving to live in an institution

"I was small when I came [to Echoing Hills], I was about 9 or 10. I came here to learn to do everything on my own. My dad and my mum made the decision to bring me here. They had visited other places but did not take me to them. When I came here I felt happy. Me, I am a happy girl, when I was small I felt happy, and still, now I am a woman I feel happy to be here."

Accessing education

"I went to school when I was small and then when I was 13 or 14 I went to school at Bilingual [a mainstream school near Echoing Hills]. Because I was new they sent me to class 2 [this would have been several years behind the appropriate class for Maame Yaa's chronological age]. I went to school for a while and then I dropped because of the way they are treating people like me. Some of them were laughing at me. Some of them said they did not like me to come near them. They think the disability will affect them. They think they will get it. If I am going out in a group they sometimes don't want me to go – I should leave them and not go. I can walk but I have to take my time. I went on vacation break from school and did not go back. They should be helpful, they should do us good, they should help us. Here [at Echoing Hills] they are more helpful. Everyone can learn."

Societal views and impact on sense of self-worth

"We are human beings. [To] those people who think we are not human beings, [I say] we are human being like them, so they should be careful before they say with their mouth. One day it will come to them [and they will realise], we are human beings, it's all by God's grace we are alive."

"Disability is not inability. We can do things on our own. My mum told me that and the people around told me. My brothers and sisters liked me. You should not try to kill yourself because of the disability."

Causes of disability

"It's not anything. It's God who gives me intellectual disability. He likes how I am. He told me. No, it's not a curse. If you think disability is a curse, then why has it happened to me and not to you? It's not us – it's something that has happened. It's the devil who makes us believe [that it's a curse]. It's not anything that they say in this world. God loves me and he loves everyone."

Dreams and ambitions

"I want to be a carer. I like to help people. With a helping hand, I can help people with disabilities and able people too.

[Although I have a disability] I can do things that other people can't do. Sometimes if I am there and if a place is dirty, I can do it [clean]. I can see. I used to feed Small Kofi when he came here. I have been feeding him small, small. He now knows how to eat on his own. I will help him to do it, if I am not there I will ask someone to help him. I try to help all people with disabilities to do things on their own. I help them to sweep, to do cleaning, the rest of the things.

My dream for my life is to be working, to get a work [a paid job] and someone to get to marry me and after the wedding to work, to get all that I need. I think it's good for people with disabilities to get married, to get someone by your side, it's good and to have a child. Some people are telling me I should get married. But I don't think it is now [it is not yet time].

I would be comfortable living in my own house. I want to live in my own house with my own things. I am learning things so I can do things to live on my own."

Gloria's story: "People did not believe I could do that but I am doing it"

Gloria was born in 1987 and was 31 at the time of writing. She lives in Pedu, just outside Cape Coast, with her mother and her 28-year-old sister. She was born in Accra, but after about five months moved to the Pedu area. She says her disability is cerebral palsy and her intellectual ability "is not good enough to do things I would have liked to do, like becoming a lawyer".

Access to education at a NGO-run special school

"When I was about 5, I started going to St Elisabeth's [a NGO-run special school and home for children], as a day pupil. It is a school not far from Pedu. There were many children. I had some friends at school, there. It was good being there. I liked the school. I liked cooking there and learnt English there too. We learnt to make doormats from rag pieces. The doormats were sold from the school.

At my school, I didn't like a teacher who insulted us, Madam. Not the head teacher. Every day Madam would say 'Gloria is a bad girl, ooo'. I did not like it. She was not joking. When it became too much, I will isolate myself and after a while someone would call me to come and join my friends.

One day I got annoyed with Madam, and said to her 'What is this. I don't like that, Madam, I am a good person'. She said it was not like that. But she did not change her behaviour and continued to insult me and other pupils.

Some of my friends have now given birth [without being married]. I am not like that. I don't follow men. So how do you say a person like that is a bad girl?

I liked going the beach from school in the school bus. Just a few of the pupils will go. We would go to a beach every month. Madam who insulted me used to come too but I managed."

"I did not see my school friends in the holidays as they lived a long way away.

I had one friend living round here called Amina who is still my friend.

My sister went to a normal school, Pedu School, near our home."

Learning skills to start her own business

"I used to help my mother with her fruit selling when I was at home and in the holidays. I learnt how to do trading by working with my mum.

I would have liked to become a lawyer but I did not get the chance. I stayed on at St Elisabeth's, helping there, till I was 25 and I continued to visit the school to help there, until I opened my shop recently. They gave me money to help me start the shop."

Views on disability

"I know people see me as disabled, but I can do many things. I am also a Ghanaian, I am also a human being. Customers come to the shop thinking they will be able to cheat me because of my disability, but no one can cheat me."

"I don't have problems in my family, my mother loves me and my sister loves me. And my brother also likes me so much because he likes me always being frank."

Views on causes and treatment of disability

Gloria attends a Methodist church with her mother.

"I don't get involved in activities at the church apart from the service. I don't want any trouble. I know who I am so I don't involve myself. I like church – I like the drums there. No one at church says that I should be healed of my disability. I have accepted that I have a disability. Whatever you do the condition will not go. That is how God made me. I have had people saying they would pray for me to be healed at other churches. But I have accepted I have a disability."

Dreams and aspirations

"I would like my shop to get big. I would like to be a good girl and help others with intellectual disabilities through advocacy. I would like to get married and have children, but not in a rush way. I want to take my time. If you do not exercise patience and go after men, and make a wrong choice, coming back will be a problem.

I would like to continue as a self-advocate to help other people with intellectual disabilities be treated better. I want people to know that being disabled does not mean you are mad. Many disabled people are in a much worse situation than me – I have been able to open and run a shop, people did not believe I could do that but I am doing it. So, I want to tell everyone that people with disabilities can do things."

Conclusion

Maame Yaa and Gloria are positive examples of Ghanaians who have been able to overcome some of the challenges their label has brought them, to maintain and build confidence in themselves, and to have positive aspirations for the future. The twentieth century may have seen little change for people in Ghana, as societal attitudes – particularly in relation to rights – remained largely unchanged. However, the positive example of these two women demonstrates that, despite the huge challenges facing people, and their families, there is hope for a brighter future, through a combination of self-advocacy and continuing pressure from parents and supporters to drive positive changes in social attitudes and priorities.

Notes

[1] See 'Opening the doors to justice for persons with intellectual disabilities in Ghana', a booklet by Inclusion Ghana (2013, available at: www.inclusion-ghana.org/resources/brochures/DRF%20Booklet.pdf). This is aimed at the general public and professionals, and states on p 12: 'The following do not cause intellectual disabilities; curses, spiritual forces, witchcraft, punishment, contact with a person with an intellectual disability'. It seeks to address widely held beliefs in Ghana.

[2] PACID (Ghana), the earliest parent group for persons with intellectual disability of which we are aware, was founded by Mrs Salome Francois in 2001, based at New Horizon Special School in Accra. It was initially funded by DSI, Denmark (The Danish Council of Organizations of Disabled People) to give support to parents and guardians of children with an intellectual disability in Ghana and also to advocate for policies and programmes that serve their interest. PACID is made up of parents and guardians together with relevant professionals. (Interview with Mrs Francois, 2017, and information from PACID website: www.newhorizon-school-gh.com/pacid-ghana.html [accessed 28/1/2018]).

References

Agbenyega, J. (2003) 'The power of labelling discourse in the construction of disability in Ghana'. A paper presented at the Australian Association of Research in Education Conference, in Newcastle, December 2003.

Al Jazeera (2013) 'Spirit Child (Ghana)'. Available at: https://impact.gijn.org/case-studies/spirit–child-ghana/ (downloaded 28/1/2018).

Anthony, J.H. (2010) 'Towards inclusion: influences of culture and internationalisation on personhood, educational access, policy and provision for students with autism in Ghana'. Doctoral thesis, University of Sussex. Available at: sro.sussex.ac.uk/2347

Baffoe, M. (2013) 'Stigma, discrimination and marginalization: gateways to oppression of persons with disabilities in Ghana, West Africa', *Journal of Educational and Social Research*, 3(1): 187–98.

BBC (2015) 'The worst country in the world to be disabled?', first broadcast BBC3, July 2015. Part of the Defying the Label season. Executive producer Alison Gregory; presenter Sophie Morgan.

Hervie, V.M. (2013) 'Shut up! Social inclusion of children with intellectual disabilities in Ghana'. Master's thesis, Faculty of Social Sciences, University of Nordland, Norway. Available at: http://hdl.handle.net/11250/139975

Nukunya, G.K. (2003) *Tradition and change in Ghana: An introduction to sociology* (second edition), Accra: Ghana Universities Press.

FIVE

A Greek Neverland: the history of the Leros asylums' inmates with intellectual disability (1958–95)

Danae Karydaki

All children, except one, grow up.
Barrie, 1911, 3

Introduction

On 10 September 1989, a Greek scandal made headlines in the British *Observer* newspaper; the article's title was 'Europe's Guilty Secret' and the front page depicted several naked male mental patients looking desperate, wandering around the Leros Psychiatric Hospital buildings in Lepida. The piece described the appalling living conditions under which the patients struggled to survive for years. 'Hundreds of mentally ill and handicapped men, women and children,' it read, 'have been left to rot in concentration camp conditions on a remote Greek island. The full horror of the plight of the lost souls on the Aegean island of Leros, 172 miles south-east from the mainland port of Piraeus, is revealed today after two *Observer* journalists gained access to the hospital' (Merritt, 1989a, 1989b).

This 'guilty secret' had in fact been known in Greece long before 1989. A group of young Leros doctors and deinstitutionalisation activists had presented the situation in a Greek-French symposium on social psychiatry, organised by the renowned psychiatrist and psychoanalyst Panayotis Sakellaropoulos in December 1981 (Sakellaropoulos, 1984, 1990). An article about Leros accompanied by disturbing pictures had appeared on the front page of *Eleftherotypia*, one of the most widely circulated newspapers in the country, as early as June 1983 (*Leriaka Nea*, 1983; *Eleftherotypia*, 1983). Also in 1983, the newly elected socialist government had introduced Law 1397 providing for the creation of the Greek National Health System, which included Article 21 providing for the organisation and reform of psychiatric services, while in 1984 it even managed to receive 'exceptional financial support in favour of Greece in the social field' from the European Community, based on EEC Regulation 815/84 (*Government Gazette*, 1983; *Official Journal of the European Communities*, 1984). As the French philosopher Félix Guattari (2015, p 50) notes in his Leros diaries in October 1989, 'the *Observer* journalist had to look for old pictures for his piece, since Pavilion 16, some sort of 'snake pit' [*fosse aux serpents*], where 165 patients, naked and crammed like cattle, lived for years, does not exist any more.' No matter how distorted, delayed, provocative or voyeuristic the *Observer* representation of Leros might have been, however, it did make 1989 into a turning point in the history of Greek psychiatry: the international publicity triggered by the *Observer* article that illustrated the Leros asylums as a European disgrace opened the way for the deinstitutionalisation of Leros and the long-overdue reform of Greek psychiatry.

What often goes unnoticed, however, is that among the Leros asylums' inmates were also numerous people with intellectual disability. 'The smell,' wrote Merritt (1989b) in the *Observer*, 'hits like the reek of an abattoir and the scenes flicker past like some depraved peep show. No distinction is made between mental illness and mental disability.' British psychiatrists John Henderson and Bob Grove (1999), who were involved in monitoring the reform programme for the European Commission, noted respectively that the patient population in the Leros Psychiatric Hospital (henceforth LPH) was 'an admixture of those with a psychiatric diagnosis and also those with a diagnosis of what is still known in most of Europe as "mental retardation"'. Some of these inmates with intellectual disability were accommodated in the LPH along with patients suffering from mental disorders, whereas others, some under age, lived in a separate unit, the Institution for Misfit[1] Children of Leros (known as Leros PIKPA Asylum).

The story of these people, who present an emblematic paradigm in the history of intellectual disability in Greece and elsewhere, has yet to be told. Historians of intellectual disability have largely focused their research on Western English-speaking countries, such as Britain and the USA (see Trent, 1994; Wright and Digby, 1996; Jackson, 2000; Wright, 2001; McDonagh, 2008). Greece is a relatively small country at the crossroads of East and West and nearly all its archival material regarding intellectual disability is only accessible by Greek-speaking researchers. Thus, apart from some notable exceptions (Ploumbidis, 1981; Gonela et al, 2000; Kritsotaki, 2016), the history of intellectual disability in Greece has, so far, been largely neglected by historians. This chapter aims to trace and historicise the unexplored practices and policies towards people with intellectual disability at the Leros asylums between 1958, when the LPH opened its gates, and 1995, when the first attempt at the deinstitutionalisation of the Leros asylums was completed. I place emphasis on how people with intellectual disability were mistreated and socially excluded by being abandoned to live under inhumane living conditions on a remote island while being, at the same time, infantilised in the discourse of mental health professionals, policy-makers and, at times, fellow inmates. In so doing, not only does this chapter shed light on an issue neglected by historians but also, and most importantly, attempts to complement an international perspective of the history of intellectual disability.

Island of Outcasts

'In ancient Greece,' a European delegate is quoted by the *Observer*, 'the entrance to Hades was in a cave on the Peloponnese peninsula. In modern Greece, it is on Leros' (Merritt, 1989a). Leros has a long history as 'home' for those excluded by Greek society and, at times, also abused by the Greek state. In 1912, Leros passed from the Ottomans to the Italians and, during the inter-war period, it became 'Italy's most important and heavily fortified naval base', accommodating more than 7,000 Italian troops in Lepida near the town of Porto Lago in Lakki (Doumanis, 1997, 45). After the 1947 Peace Treaty, the Dodecanese were ceded to Greece. In the wake of the Greek Civil War, fought between the victorious right-wing National Greek army (backed by the UK and the USA) and the defeated military branch of the Greek Communist Party (supported by the Soviet Union), the former military bases on Leros acquired a new use: as a technical school and re-education institution for young communists and delinquents between 14 and 21 years old, under the name 'Royal Technical School of Leros' (Danforth and Van Boeschoten, 2012, 100–102). Some years later, during the military junta (1967–74), the same infrastructure was transformed into internment camps for political dissidents (*The New York Times*, 1970). For the greatest part of their history, however, these buildings accommodated mentally ill and intellectually disabled inmates.

On 7 May 1957, the LPH, initially called 'Psychopaths' Colony of Leros', was established through a Royal Decree by the conservative government of Konstantinos Karamanlis (*Government Gazette*, 1957) and the first patients were transferred there in early 1958. Its establishment was based on Law 6077 of 1934 providing for the organisation of public mental hospitals, and it fell under the administration of the Ministry of State Hygiene and Perception (later to be renamed Ministry of Health). Indeed, the policy of the LPH to admit both people suffering from mental disorders and people with intellectual disability was also based on Law 6077: Article 1 determined that the purpose for the establishment of public mental hospitals in Greece was the treatment and care of 'psychopaths, epileptics, alcoholics, heavily perverted and mentally retarded persons' (*Government Gazette*, 1934, 457).[2]

The inspiration for a 'Psychopaths' Colony' on the remote island of Leros was drawn from Article 4 of the same law, which provided for the creation of 'rural psychopaths' colonies' where patients were expected to work in farming activities (*Government Gazette*, 1934, 458). As perhaps hinted by the term 'colony', and legally grounded on Legislative Decree 2592 of 1953 on using mental hospitals to serve the needs of the whole country (*Government Gazette*, 1953a), the purpose of the Leros asylum was not to host the mentally ill or intellectually disabled people of the Dodecanese; it was to relieve the existing mental hospitals of big cities, overcrowded because of the terrible post-Civil War social conditions (Papadimitriou, 2013, 205).

Patients selected for transfer to Leros were those who had not been visited by their families for at least 12 months (Papadimitriou, 2013, 206) and were thus considered 'abandoned by their next of kin' or, as the psychiatrist of the Leros Hospital Ioannis Loukas put it, 'socially unclaimed' and 'mentally incurable' (Loukas, 2006). Child psychiatrist John Tsiantis, one of the protagonists of the Leros PIKPA Asylum intervention and deinstitutionalisation in the early 1990s, and his partners argued that the stigma and shame brought to families, along with health professionals' opinion that the patients 'were indiscriminately not worth the effort or the concern', made families abandon their intellectually disabled members to various institutions (Tsiantis et al, 2000). Abandonment by family is also connected to a widely accepted historiographical view that the reason behind the invention of the 19th-century asylum in Western Europe was the rapid social changes that followed the rise of capitalist economy. Families could no longer take care of their mentally ill or intellectually disabled members because breadwinners had to work outside of the household (Scull, 1977; Jay, 2016, 99–100). Greece had a more traditional social structure than other European countries but, as historian Efi Avdela (2002, 2013) has argued, in the post-Civil War period Greek society was gradually modernising, and the Greek family was experiencing significant changes, such as urbanisation and the spread of women's work outside of the home (Kritsotaki, 2018). These changes perhaps also explain why families, otherwise so fundamental to the Greek social fabric, chose to send their intellectually disabled members to Leros in the late 1950s. The psychiatrist Dimitris Ploumbidis (1981, 108), who was also later involved with the Leros deinstitutionalisation project, notes accordingly that the presence of people with intellectual disability in mental hospitals is a sign of 'disintegration of traditional society'; this is why, he observes, evidence shows that there were very few people with intellectual disability among mental hospitals' inmates in the Greek-speaking areas of the Ottoman Empire in the early twentieth century.

The case of Leros – which, because of both geography and distance from urban centres, resembles a natural prison – is crucial in the context of this chapter because it illustrates the practice of excluding, excommunicating and, indeed, keeping the greatest possible physical distance from people with intellectual disability in the mid-20th century. Psychiatrist Theodoros Megalooikonomou (2016, 149), one of the pioneers of the Leros deinstitutionalisation movement in the 1990s, attempts to describe this exclusion of the undesirables on the island of Leros in social terms:

> Leros … has been used, throughout the 20th century … as a space of stoppage and counterweight of the Greek society's internal class contradictions or, otherwise, as a place of exile and concentration of 'social waste' of any kind. These contradictions appear in the everyday function of a complicated social system that constantly and inherently produces and reproduces various groups of excluded, pariahs and outcasts, performing against them what [the Italian psychiatry reformer] Franco Basaglia called 'peace crimes' (crimini di pace).

The Law 6077 of 1934 that enforced both the accommodation of people with intellectual disability together with the mentally ill and the creation of 'rural psychopaths' colonies' away from the urban centres allowed for Leros to be turned into a bin for what Megalooikonomou calls 'social waste'. In this way, Leros inmates with intellectual disability became an inherent part of Greece's 'social waste', of those who, as the French anthropologist Claude Levi-Strauss (1961, 386) observed, were vomited out of the community.

The fact that among those considered 'social waste' in mid-20th-century Greece were also people with intellectual disability contributes to a broader debate about whether people with intellectual disability have always been considered unwelcome by the community. More specifically, Simon Jarrett (2015) critically revisited the historical senses of 'community' and argued that before the emergence of the asylum, people with intellectual disability had naturally been included in the social structure. 'It is exclusion therefore,' he writes, 'that is the anomalous exception in historical terms, and the idea of inclusion is not a modern paradigm shift imagined by late-twentieth-century reforming advocates but represents rather a return to a societal norm.' Indeed, in the case of Greece, Ploumbidis (1981, 3) observes that before Greece was declared an independent state in the 19th century, intellectually disabled people were not locked up in institutions: some of them were highly respected and even granted impunity on the grounds of certain religious beliefs.

As years went by, the living conditions in the LPH were getting worse, while the population was increasing (Bairaktaris, 2007, 133). Ioannis Loukas (2017, personal communication) first went to Leros in 1981 on placement and then returned in 1988 to train for his speciality in psychiatry. He recalls how the Leros inmates survived under the most extreme conditions of asylum life, inside military barracks, in wards consisting of 90–180 people. In Pavilion 11, 1,100 patients of mixed diagnosis (ie including people with intellectual disability) lived next to each other, 'with no space or time for themselves, as part of a mass or a herd, with no individual identity, with no human rights, and with social death as the sole prospect ahead of them' (Loukas, 2006; 2017, personal communication). The late leftist activist and Leros Hospital psychiatrist Efi Skliri (2015, 8, 12), who went to Leros to do her placement after having studied in Germany, wrote in her diary in 1979 that the LPH was 'neither a mental hospital nor an asylum or a prison and, of course, not even a purgatory'. It was, as she characteristically notes, 'Dachau', one of the most commonly used metaphors, together with 'Auschwitz', for illustrating human atrocities towards fellow humans.

Life story 1: Dimitris*

Dimitris was born in 1963 in a small Greek town. His father left Greece and went to work as an immigrant in another country. Dimitris stayed with his mother and two sisters and, at some point, moved to Athens. When he was 10 years old, his mother sent him away to a big psychiatric hospital in Athens. In 1980, when he was 17 years old, he was sent to Leros to be locked up in the LPH. "Back then, did they tell you why they brought you here?" Dimitris is asked by a journalist in Jane Gabriel's Channel 4 documentary 'Island of Outcasts' (Gabriel, 1990).

"No, they didn't tell me anything," he replies. Seven years after his admission to the LPH and 14 after his first admission to a mental hospital, he was diagnosed with mild intellectual disability. Even the unskilled guards at the time thought he should not have been living in an asylum as he was fully functional and capable of working 'in the outside world'.

Since the deinstitutionalisation of Leros, Dimitris has been living in an apartment outside the LPH along with members of the nursing staff and other inmates who were ready for their 'social reintegration'. Everybody on the island knows him and speaks highly of him. He has also been working in the Lakki port where the boats dock for many years.

He says that in the institution he dreamt of watching television, drinking coffee (which was not allowed) and going back home to live with his mother in Athens. He has spoken of his dream of marriage: "This woman I'll marry, she will only be mine. I will pay all her expenses. I will pay the rent, I will be washing her clothes, I will be cooking for her whatever she wants. She will have her wine, a nice bed and we'll be sleeping together, hugging, every night."

Dimitris, a person with mild intellectual disability whose mother sent him to Leros during his adolescence for no obvious medical reason, like so many others at the time in Greece, never went back home, except for a few times to visit his sisters. "Where do you like it most? Athens or here?" I ask him in the present day. "Athens," he mouths (he recently had a tracheotomy), "but here is also nice." Despite the traumatic experience of his exclusion, Dimitris is now an equal member of the Leros community.

* Dimitris is a pseudonym of an LPH inmate who told me his story.

Forever children

The LPH was not the only place that accommodated people with intellectual disability on Leros. In 1961, the PIKPA Asylum also opened its gates on the island. This was part of a large network of institutions that belonged to the Patriotic Institution for Social Welfare and Perception.[3] It was founded in 1914 as a ladies' charity under the name 'Patriotic Association of Greek Women', and its resources included members' contributions, donations, royal sponsorship and state funding. During the inter-war period, it emerged as the main institution of social policy and practice for maternity and childhood.

At a time when child mortality was still very high in Greece it used a large network of female volunteers to enlighten working-class mothers on issues of hygiene and normal development of children (Theodorou, 2015, 82–5). In 1929, the institution, under its new name the 'Patriotic Institution for Child Protection', was exclusively oriented to the promotion of child welfare, and in 1936 it was renamed the 'Patriotic Institution for Social Welfare and Perception' (PIKPA). According to Mandatory Law 1950, issued in 1939 (*Government Gazette*, 1939), the Patriotic Institution for Social Welfare and Perception was based in Athens and was also, like the LPH, under the auspices of the Ministry of State Hygiene and Perception. Although other aims were recorded, such as care for the poor and victims of natural disasters, its principal cause was to protect maternity and childhood. This is manifested, for example, in the organisation of the first Balkan Exhibition for Child Protection that was held in Athens in April 1936 (Hellenic Literary and Historical Archive [ELIA], 1936).

In 1953, Legislative Decree 2690 (*Government Gazette*, 1953b) allowed the formation of PIKPA services for the protection of maternity and childhood in the country and a few years later, in March 1961 the PIKPA Asylum of Leros was launched under the name 'Leros Centre for Child Care', through Royal Decree 147 of 1961. As in the case of the LPH, Leros was chosen because of its infrastructure; an Italian building in Lakki that was later transformed into the Royal School of Housekeeping for teenage girls became the base of the PIKPA Asylum. Its purpose was to care for children between 0 and 18 years old 'suffering from incurable physical handicaps ... severe non-trainable mental retardations and, in general, incurable and non-improvable severe disorders with or without neurological and physical damage' (*Government Gazette*, 1961). Again, the Leros PIKPA Asylum was not exclusively designed for people with intellectual disability. However, when John Tsiantis's medical team assessed the PIKPA Asylum inmates in 1991, all of them were diagnosed as 'mentally retarded' while many also had some physical impairment such as motor impairment or blindness; 55% of them presented 'profound mental retardation', 25% 'severe mental retardation', and 20% 'moderate to mild mental retardation' (Tsiantis, 1995).

Like the rest of the inmates of the island, PIKPA Asylum inmates were 'effectively sequestered from their families and society at large' (Tsiantis, 1995). Their physical and social living conditions were as horrific as those of the LPH, if not worse: they lived in a 1930s military building with no lifts or ramps for the physically disabled; toilets and showers were only introduced a few years before the beginning of the deinstitutionalisation project and were not covered by the inadequate central heating of the building; and they ate (or were fed) in bed. Many were routinely confined to bed by force when staff were unable to enforce discipline (Tsiantis et al, 1995). John Henderson (1995) describes the impact that these living conditions had on mental health professionals in the late 1980s: 'Nor will anyone who saw them ever forget the tragic sight of naked boys and girls crawling about or lying on dirty coarse blankets spread upon the bare floors of their wards, or those who were so terribly deformed and misshapen lying so still in their beds as to appear lifeless.' Even after completion of the first stage of deinstitutionalisation, in June 1995, when there was a 'calmer atmosphere everywhere' on Leros, the British mental health professional and former president of the World Federation for Mental Health Edith Morgan wrote in her personal notes that there was no play material or staff stimulation for those lying in their beds (Morgan, 1995).

Life story 2: Ioanna*

Ioanna formerly lived in the Leros PIKPA Asylum and, during the 1990s deinstitutionalisation programme, was transferred to the guesthouse 'Thetis' in Athens. She was born out of wedlock in largely conservative 1960s Greece. She was separated from her mother at birth and put into the custody of the Patriotic Institution for Social Welfare and Perception (PIKPA). Between the ages of 1 and 7, she was taken to live with a foster family. Her foster mother rejected her, and she was admitted to the Leros PIKPA Asylum.

She moved to the guesthouse in Athens in 1993 at the age of 30, and was diagnosed with moderate intellectual disability profoundly affected by chronic institutionalisation. Medical reports from PIKPA describe her as adequately functional but with frequent outbursts of anger and aggression, often withdrawn, and with signs of depression. She hardly communicated with staff, had no family contact, and her vocabulary was particularly poor.

On moving to the Athens guesthouse she kept repeating to herself "I've got no mother and no father". Staff decided to track down Ioanna's mother through social services. It was found that the mother too appeared to have a moderate intellectual disability, had lived in a nursing home since birth, and had become pregnant through a rape. A series of meetings were held with both the mother and Ioanna, eventually leading to them meeting together for the first time since Ioanna's birth (her mother believed she had given birth to a boy). They have established regular telephone contact since then. Ioanna now tells everyone where she comes from. She approaches the staff to say "I've got a name" and persistently asks when her name day is. She has grown more interested in what is happening around her, built relationships with members of the staff and other residents, has sung in front of an audience and become interested in her appearance and her body.

Ioanna's story is indicative of the excommunication and intergenerational violation of the rights of people with intellectual disability in 20th-century Greece. But it is also indicative of how deinstitutionalisation and family reunification can prove a reparatory experience.

* This story is extracted from a secondary source (Loukakos, 2003), and the name is used in accordance with the authors' choice.

The relevance of the origins of the Leros PIKPA Asylum to our discussion is that PIKPA's historically manifested aim to promote child protection and ensure child care resonates with how often the Leros inmates with intellectual disability were treated or referred to as 'children'. "We called them 'paidakia' [small children]," Charis Evangellou, a former technician at the LPH, and Maria X, a nurse, told me (2018, personal communication). The infantilisation of the Leros inmates with intellectual disability had an institutional as well as a discursive aspect.

Regarding the institutional aspect of infantilisation, firstly, because of its history as a women's charity for maternity and child protection, the PIKPA branch of Leros administratively belonged to the Ministry of Health sector of welfare, unlike the LPH, which administratively belonged to the Ministry of Health sector of mental health. Precisely for this reason, its deinstitutionalisation was delayed because the EEC Regulation 815/84 was initially designed to cover only mental hospitals (Tsiantis, 1994). Secondly, although the Leros PIKPA Asylum was legally bound by Royal Decree 147 of 1961 to accommodate children and adolescents, many of its inmates continued to live there long after they turned 18. 'At the start of the project in February 1991,' wrote John Tsiantis, 'the PIKPA institution housed 165 residents, aged between 8 and 46 years, living in excessive dependence under appalling physical and social conditions in a totally depersonalized environment characterized by deprivation and almost total lack of stimulation' (Tsiantis et al, 2000). Ann Gath, registrar of Britain's Royal College of Psychiatrists between 1988 and 1993, who visited the Leros PIKPA Asylum in May 1991, writes that at the time of her visit only 31 inmates were younger than 18. Despite their actual age, reports Gath, they were 'often referred to as children' (Gath, 1992). John Henderson (1995) observed:

> No one who visited the PIKPA institution at that time could ever forget the appalling physical and social living conditions which over 160 *so-called children* and the staff had to endure. Most of these *children* had grown to adolescence or adulthood during their years of incarceration. (Emphasis added)

Both Gath and Henderson underline the fact that the PIKPA inmates were referred to or called 'children', although they were adults. This kind of discourse resonates with the practice of infantilisation of people with intellectual disabilities, which was applied both to the PIKPA inmates and the intellectually disabled inmates of the LPH. In June 1979, when Efi Skliri was working at the LPH, she wrote in her diary of an instance when infantilisation of the Leros inmates with intellectual disability, in this case, a person with microcephaly, was uncannily intertwined with feelings one may develop towards juvenile pets:

> He truly does not seem like hurting, what the hell. I'll soon come to believe that madmen don't hurt, as it is the prevalent view here in Dachau, although I propagandise that they can neither convey it in words nor with facial expression. I give [them] candies, and N, a person with microcephalia, whom [the other inmates] obsessively drag into being naughty,[4] asks me if I love him. At that point, I broke out. I tenderly caressed his monstrous head and told him I adore him. It is barbaric, all these people being there and me not being able to build a relationship with them, one that I would do with kittens (Skliri, 2015, 16).

In this case, Skliri offers candies to people suffering from mental illness while wondering, almost in existential dread, why she cannot build a caring relationship with them or feel as she would towards baby animals, why the patients are so dehumanised that they are often perceived as not feeling any pain. She finally breaks out before the person with microcephalia and intellectual disability whom she sees as innocent, dragged into 'sin' by the others, echoing what James

Trent (1994: 10) described as the image of 'feeble-minded people' as 'children of pure nature' in 18th-century America. At that moment, Skliri adopts a maternal role after his somewhat childish question of whether she loves him, verbally confirms her love, and caresses him as if he were a child.

This maternal role was not only adopted by mental health professionals but also by fellow inmates. The psychiatrist Kaiti Karanikola said in her attempt to explain why it was appropriate, in her view, to accommodate people with intellectually disabilities in the same spaces as people with mental ill health: 'The schizophrenics help the retarded. They treat them like their own children. They have one or two of them under their protection' (Gabriel, 1990). In the context of an isolated mental hospital on a remote island, where people with intellectual disability and mentally ill patients live together, and ties with the real families are usually severed, dynamics resembling that of a family develop. In this condition, people with intellectual disabilities are usually treated as 'children'. Indeed, even after the enforcement of EEC Regulation 815/84 and the transfer of small groups of patients from Leros to guesthouses in Athens and elsewhere in the early 1990s, such dynamics were still at play. Giorgos Koutas (1994, 21) describes how in the UMHRI guesthouse in Athens, organised by Dimitris Ploumbidis, there was one female patient, T, who undertook a maternal role towards the other members of the group, among whom there was also Th, an intellectually disabled man. In her description of certain more able women inmates who undertook such a maternal role towards their fellow inmates with intellectual disability in the Indiana School, Licia Carlson (2010, 65) argues that '[t]he mothering role played by these women was in part justified by the infantilisation of the feebleminded ... [i]f all of the adults and children housed within the institution are thought of as children, then it is only natural that they need a mother to care for them'.

The infantilisation of people with intellectual disability emerges perhaps from certain behaviours brought about in the institutional environment of the Leros PIKPA Asylum that Tsiantis et al (1995) described as 'excessive dependence and inhibition'. In his account of lay attitudes towards 'idiots' in Victorian England, David Wright (1996, 124) observes that 'the [intellectual] disability of the individual evoked strong allusions to the permanency of the childlike dependence' and records relatives' testimonies who illustrate the 'idiots' with phrases such as 'childish in her ways' or 'childlike in his innocence'. People with intellectual disabilities were thus seen as dependent, helpless and in constant need of a parent. Besides, it is no coincidence that PIKPA, a women's charity, was transformed into a public institution, supposedly aimed at replacing the inadequate, unwilling or abandoning mothers of children with intellectual disabilities, or that the most important advocate for turning intellectual disability into a public concern in post-war Greece was the PanHellenic Union of Parents and Guardians of Unadjusted Children, namely a parents' movement (Kritsotaki, 2016).

There also emerges a matter of scale related to what Wright (1996: 124) described as 'the relative backwardness of the child [with intellectual disability] *vis-à-vis* other children or adolescents of the same age'. This 'backwardness' is perceived as the inability of persons with intellectual disability to reach the 'adult mind' and, thus, their fate to stay children forever. Michel Foucault (2006, 209), drawing on the work of the 19th-century French physician Édouard Séguin, also described how 'idiocy' or 'mental retardation' can philosophically be seen as the early stage of child development: 'The idiot is a certain degree of childhood, or again, if you like, childhood is a certain way of passing more or less quickly through the degrees of idiocy, debility, or mental retardation.' The Leros inmates with intellectual disability were thus perceived, referred to and, at times, treated as children.

Conclusion

Up until the early 1990s, and despite the efforts on behalf of doctors and activists to raise awareness of the issue throughout the 1980s, the Leros inmates with intellectual disabilities had indeed been, as the *Observer* title underlined, 'Europe's guilty secret'. They were abandoned, excommunicated, forced to live in appalling conditions. By the time the deinstitutionalisation project began, they had already suffered severe deprivation, extreme institutionalisation, and violation of their fundamental human rights. Their existence and their humanity were forgotten by their families, society and, above all, the Greek state.

As far as mistreatment and exclusion are concerned, people with intellectual disability were not distinguished from people who were diagnosed as mentally ill. Just as the LPH was purposed both for people with intellectual disability and for people suffering from mental disorders, so were the practices of excommunication, abandonment, neglect and abuse. What was different in the case of the Leros inmates with intellectual disability was their infantilisation in an institutional and discursive power network. Many of them continued to live in a children's hospital (Leros PIKPA Asylum) long after they had come of age, while the principal institution that supposedly ensured their welfare was a former women's charity that had for a long time been the main actor in child protection in Greece (the Patriotic Institution for Social Welfare and Perception). Moreover, the mental health professionals and, at times, some of their patients treated or referred to the Leros inmates with intellectual disability as children and apparently developed feelings one may have towards children.

Because of what has come to be known as the 'modern concept of childhood' (Ariès, 1962, 34), namely the perception of children as not merely being of a lower age but as having different qualities than adults, the infantilisation of people with intellectual disabilities makes their exclusion and abuse in the institutional context of Leros even more striking. In the modern era, a picture or report of a child victim of war, abuse or neglect evokes more powerful feelings than one of an adult in a similar situation. In her book *Precarious life: The powers of mourning and violence*, Judith Butler (2004) deals with how power signifies, defines, assesses and classifies which bodies are worthy of mourning and which ones are not; the bodies of children, or at least the bodies of children in the Western world, are perceived, in the West, as more valuable and worthy of mourning than those of adults. In this light, because the Leros inmates with intellectual disabilities were institutionally and discursively treated as children, their abused and socially excluded bodies must have been experienced as worthier of compassion and mourning. The intellectual disability is normalised or even humanised because it is attached to childhood, or as Foucault (2006: 209) put it, '[idiocy or mental retardation] are temporal varieties of stages within the normative development of the child. The idiot belongs to childhood, as previously he belonged to illness.' When Efi Skliri (2015, 16) was afraid that she would end up dehumanising her patients, she broke out when she imagined and treated N, an intellectually disabled patient, as a child in need of words of love and human touch. Infantilisation can undoubtedly function as a patronising and condescending practice towards people with intellectual disability. Nonetheless, because we do not yet inhabit a world where all bodies are worth of mourning, infantilisation may have contributed in occasional avoidance of the Leros inmates' dehumanisation because of the social and emotional charge that childhood bears. In any case, it is now up to historians of intellectual disability to further explore the history of this Greek Neverland, where some children never grew up.

Notes

[1] Instead of 'misfit', the word 'unadjusted' has recently been suggested as an alternative translation for the Greek word 'απροσάρμοστα' (see Kritsotaki, 2016).

2   Unless otherwise indicated, translations from Greek are my own.
3   PIKPA [ΠΙΚΠΑ] stands for the initials of the institution in Greek: Πατριωτικό Ίδρυμα Κοινωνικής Πρόνοιας και Αντιλήψεως.
4   The expression 'drag him into being naughty' is used here as the best possible translation for the phrase 'τον πονηρεύουν' which bears a sexual connotation.

References

Ariès, P. (1962) *Centuries of childhood: A social history of family life*, trs R. Baldick. New York: Alfred A. Knopf.

Avdela, E. (2002) *Δια λόγους τιμής: Βία, συναισθήματα και αξίες σε μια μετεμφυλιακή Ελλάδα [For reasons of honour: Violence, emotions, and values in post-Civil War Greece]*, Athens: Nefeli.

Avdela, E. (2013) *'Νέοι εν κινδύνω': επιτήρηση, αναμόρφωση και δικαιοσύνη ανηλίκων μετά τον πόλεμο ['Youth at risk': Juvenile surveillance, reformation and justice after the war]*, Athens: Polis.

Bairaktaris, K. (2007) *Ψυχική Υγεία και Κοινωνική Παρέμβαση: εμπειρίες, συστήματα, πολιτικές [Mental health and social intervention: Experiences, systems, policies]*, Athens: Enallaktikes Ekdoseis.

Barrie, J.M. (1911) *Peter Pan (Peter and Wendy)*, London: Hodder & Stoughton.

Butler, J. (2004) *Precarious life: The powers of mourning and violence*, London: Verso.

Carlson, L. (2010) *The faces of intellectual disability: Philosophical reflections.* Bloomington/Indianapolis: Indiana University Press.

Danforth, L.M. and Van Boeschoten, R. (2012) *Children of the Greek Civil War: Refugees and the politics of memory*, Chicago/London: The University of Chicago Press.

Doumanis, N. (1997) *Myth and memory in the Mediterranean: Remembering fascism's empire*, London: Palgrave Macmillan.

Eleftherotypia (1983) 'Ψυχιατρείο Λέρου: Εδώ αφήστε κάθε ελπίδα ['Leros Psychiatric Hospital: here leave all your hope'], 19 June.

Foucault, M. (2006) *Psychiatric power: Lectures at the Collège de France 1973–74*, trs G. Burchell, Basingstoke/New York: Palgrave Macmillan.

Gabriel, J. (1990) 'Island of Outcasts', Channel 4.

Gath, A. (1992) 'A visit to Romania in October 1990 and to Leros in May 1991', *Journal of Intellectual Disability Research*, 36, pp 3–5.

Gonela, E., Rigopoulou, T. and Trantou, K. (2000) 'Η προσφορά του Κώστα Καλαντζή στην Ειδική Αγωγή' ['The contribution of Kostas Kalantzis to special education'], *Special Education Issues*, 10.

Government Gazette (1934) 'Νόμος 6077 περί οργανώσεως Δημόσιων Ψυχιατρίων' ['Law 6077 for the organisation of public mental hospitals]', 21 February, pp 457–64.

Government Gazette (1939) 'Αναγκαστικός Νόμος 1950/1939 περι οργανώσεως του Πατριωτικού Ιδρύματος Κοινωνικής Πρόνοιας και Αντιλήψεως' ['Mandatory Law 1950/1939 for the organisation of the Patriotic Institution for Social Welfare and Perception'], 7 September, pp 2473–6.

Government Gazette (1953a) 'Νομοθετικό διάταγμα 2592 περι οργανώσεως της Ιατρικής αντιλήψεως' ['Legislative Decree 2592 for the organisation of medical perception'], 18 September, pp 1749–55.

Government Gazette (1953b) 'Νομοθετικό διάταγμα 2690 περι συγκροτήσεως παρά των Πατριωτικό Ιδρυμάτι Κ.Π.Α. υπηρεσίας προστασίας μητρότητος και βρέφους εις την ύπαιθρον χώραν. ['Legislative Decree 2690 for the formation of protection service for maternity and childhood'], 11 November, pp 2312–14.

Government Gazette (1957) 'Βασιλικό διάταγμα περι ιδρύσεως εις Λακκί Λέρου αποικίας Ψυχοπαθών υπό μορφήν Ν.Π.Δ.Δ. ['Royal Decree for the foundation of a Psychopaths' colony in Lakki, Leros in the form of Public Law Legal Person'], 7 May, p 522.

Government Gazette (1961) 'Βασιλικό διάταγμα 147 περι συμπληρώσεως του υπηρεσιακού οργανισμού του Π.Ι.Κ.Π.Α. δια της προσθήκης θέσεων της συσταθείσης ειδικής Υπηρεσίας Περιθάλψεως Παίδων εν Λέρω' ['Royal Decree 147 for the completion of the PIKPA institution through the addition of points for the established special Service for Child Care'], 13 March, pp 449–50.

Government Gazette (1983) 'Νόμος 1397 Εθνικό Σύστημα Υγείας ['Law 1397 National Health System'], 7 October, pp 2229–2245.

Guattari, F. (2015) *Από τη Λέρο στη Λα Μπόρντ [From Leros to La Borde]*. Translated by E. Kouki. Athens: Koukkida.

Henderson, J. (1995) 'Foreword', *British Journal of Psychiatry*, 167(suppl. 28), pp. 5–6.

Henderson, J. and Grove, B. (1999) 'Leros – Escape into Life', *A Life in the Day*, 3(2), pp 5–10.

Jackson, M. (2000) *The borderland of imbecility: Medicine, society and the fabrication of the feeble mind in late Victorian and Edwardian England*, Manchester: Manchester University Press.

Jarrett, S. (2015) 'The meaning of "community" in the lives of people with intellectual disabilities: an historical perspective', *International Journal of Developmental Disabilities*, 61(2), 107–12.

Jay, M. (2016) *This way madness lies: The asylum and beyond*, Thames and Hudson/The Wellcome.

Koutas, G. (1994) 'Ερευνητικό Πανεπιστημιακό Ινστιτούτο Ψυχικής Υγείας (ΕΠΙΨΥ): Τέσσερα χρόνια λειτουργείας του ξενώνα ψυχικά ασθενών στα πλαίσια του προγράμματος "Λέρος", ['University Mental Health Research Institute (UMHRI): Four years of mental patients guesthouse in the "Leros" programme'], in E. Zacharias, C. Asimopoulos, and J. Tsiantis (eds) *Η ψυχιατρική μεταρρύθμιση στην Ελλάδα: Ξενώνες προγράμματος 'Λέρος' κανονισμός 815/84 της Ευρωπαϊκής Ένωσης, Πρακτικά [The Greek psychiatric reform: mental patients guesthouses of the 'Leros' programme, EU regulation 815/84, Proceedings]*, Athens: Ministry of Health and Welfare, pp 19–24.

Kritsotaki, D. (2016) 'Turning private concerns into public issues: mental retardation and the parents' movement in post-war Greece, c. 1950–80', *Journal of Social History*, 49(4), 982–98.

Kritsotaki, D. (2018) 'From "social aid" to "social psychiatry": mental health and social welfare in post-war Greece (1950s–1960s)', *Palgrave Communications*, 4, 9.

Leriaka Nea (1983) 'Ιδού η τουριστική προβολή του νησιού μας από την "Κυριακάτικη Ελευθεροτυπία", ['Here's the touristic promotion of our island from "Kyriakatiki Eleftherotypia"'], June, pp 1–3.

Levi-Strauss, C. (1961) *Tristes Tropiques*, trs J. Russell, New York: Criterion Books.

Loukakos, A. (2003) *Λέρος: η ελευθερία είναι θεραπευτική [Leros: Freedom is curative]*. Documentary.

Loukas, I. (2006) 'Λέρος και Ψυχιατρική Μεταρρύθμιση: Από τον Ιδρυματισμό στον Νεοϊδρυματισμό' ['Leros and psychiatric reform: from institutionalization to neo-institutionalization'], *Society and Mental Health*, 3: 26–36.

McDonagh, P. (2008) *Idiocy: A cultural history*, Liverpool: Liverpool University Press.

Megalooikonomou, T. (2016) *Λέρος: Μια ζωντανή αμφισβήτηση της Κλασικής Ψυχιατρικής [Leros: A living challenge to classical psychiatry]*, Athens: Agra.

Merritt, J. (1989a) 'Europe's guilty secret', *The Observer*, 10 September, p 1.

Merritt, J. (1989b) 'The naked and the damned', *The Observer*, 10 September, p 17.

Morgan, E. (1995) 'Edith Morgan's Diary, 14 June 1995, EDM/8/6/2/16', in *Edith Morgan Papers*, London: Wellcome Library.

Official Journal of the European Communities (1984) 'Council regulation (EEC) No 815/84 of 26 March 1984 on exceptional financial support in favour of Greece in the social field [OJ : JOL_1984_088_R_0001_007]', 31 March.

Paipeti, A., Karpetis, G. and Christogiorgos, S. (1995) 'Η γέννηση της μητέρας: η επίδραση της εμπλοκής της φυσικής οικογένειας σε προγράμματα αποασυλοποίησης και αποκατάστασης. Παρουσίαση μιας περίπτωσης' ['The birth of a mother: the impact of the biological family's involvement in projects of deinstitutionalisation and rehabilitation. A case study'], in Tsiantis, J. (ed) *Τα 'παιδιά' του ΠΙΚΠΑ Λέρου [PIKPA Leros's 'children'],* Athens: Kastaniotis, pp 197–203.

Papadimitriou, M. (2013) *Η ιστορία της Παιδοψυχιατρικής στην Ελλάδα σε σχέση με τις εξελίξεις στις ευρωπαϊκές χώρες [The history of child psychiatry in Greece in comparison to European developments],* Aristotle University of Thessaloniki.

Ploumbidis, D. (1981) *Συμβολή στη μελέτη της ιστορίας της ψυχιατρικής στην Ελλάδα: η παραδοσιακή συμπεριφορά απέναντι στους ψυχοπαθείς και τα ψυχιατρικά ιδρύματα του 19ου αιώνα [Contribution to the study of history of psychiatry in Greece: The traditional behaviour towards mental patients and mental institutions of 19th century],* University of Athens.

Sakellaropoulos, P. (ed) (1984) *Ελληνογαλλικό Συμπόσιο Κοινωνικής Ψυχιατρικής Τόμος I [Greek-French Symposium of Social Psychiatry Volume I],* Athens: Kastaniotis.

Sakellaropoulos, P. (ed.) (1990) *Ελληνογαλλικό Συμπόσιο Κοινωνικής Ψυχιατρικής Τόμος II [Greek-French Symposium of Social Psychiatry Volume II],* Athens: Kastaniotis.

Scull, A. (1977) 'Madness and segregative control: the rise of the insane asylum', *Social Problems,* 24(3), 337–51.

Skliri, E. (2015) '*Ημερολόγιο Έφης Σκλήρη*' ['Diary of Efi Skliri'], *Psychiatry Notebooks,* pp 8–19.

The New York Times (1970) 'Political prisoners in Greece issue plea', 3 January, p 7.

Theodorou, V. (2015) 'Μεταβαλλόμενα πλαίσια συνάφειας μεταξύ εθελοντών, ειδικών και κράτους: το παράδειγμα του Πατριωτικού Ιδρύματος Προστασίας του Παιδιού' ['Changing contexts of relevance between volunteers, experts and the state: the example of the Patriotic Child Protection Foundation'], in Avdela, E., Exertzoglou, C. and Lyrintzis, C. (eds) *Μορφές Δημόσιας Κοινωνικότητας στην Ελλάδα του 20ου Αιώνα [Forms of public sociality in 20th-century Greece],* Rethymno: Crete University Press, pp 82–100.

Trent, J.W. (1994) *Inventing the feeble mind: A history of mental retardation in the United States,* Berkeley, Los Angeles/London: University of California Press.

Tsiantis, J. (1994) '3η Συνεδρία: Γενική Συζήτηση', in *Η ψυχιατρική μεταρρύθμιση στην Ελλάδα: Ξενώνες προγράμματος 'Λέρος' κανονισμός 815/84 της Ευρωπαϊκής Ένωσης, Πρακτικά [The Greek psychiatric reform: Mental patients guesthouses of the 'Leros' programme, EU Regulation 815/84, Proceedings]*, Athens: Ministry of Health and Welfare, pp 131–2.

Tsiantis, J. (1995) 'Introduction', *British Journal of Psychiatry*, 167(suppl 28), 7–9.

Tsiantis, J., Perakis, A., Kordoutis, P., Kolaitis, G. and Zacharias, V. (1995) 'The Leros PIKPA Asylum: Deinstitutionalisation and Rehabilitation Project', *British Journal of Psychiatry*, 167(suppl 18), 10–45.

Tsiantis, J., Diareme, S.P. and Kolaitis, G. (2000) 'The Leros PIKPA Asylum Deinstitutionalization and Rehabilitation Project: a follow-up study on care staff fears and attitudes', *Journal of Intellectual Disabilities*, 4(4), 281–92.

van der Klis, P. (1996) *Co-drivers: Reports on the Leros project*, trs J. van der Vlist, Deventer: Centre for Vocational Rehabilitation Psychiatric Hospital Brinkgreven.

Wright, D. (1996) '"Childlike in his innocence": Lay attitudes to "idiots" and "imbeciles" in Victorian England', in D. Wright and A. Digby (eds) *From idiocy to mental deficiency: Historical perspectives on people with learning disabilities*, London and New York: Routledge, pp 118–33.

Wright, D. (2001) *Mental disability in Victorian England: The Earlswood Asylum 1847–1901*, Oxford: Oxford University Press.

Wright, D. and Digby, A. (eds) (1996) *From idiocy to mental deficiency: Historical perspectives on people with learning disabilities*, London and New York: Routledge.

'Πατριωτικόν Ίδρυμα, 1η Βαλκανική Έκθεσις Προστασίας του Παιδιού' ['Patriotic Institution, 1st Balkan Exhibition for Child Protection'], EPH.02.05.003 (1936) in *Hellenic Literary and Historical Archive [ELIA]*, Athens.

SIX

Intellectual disability in Hong Kong: then and now

Phyllis King Shui Wong

Introduction

This chapter explores policy and practice in Hong Kong, and their impact on people with intellectual disabilities and their families, in three phases: before the 1990s ('Early developments'); pre- and post-resuming sovereignty over Hong Kong ('The Golden Era'); and from the Millennium to the present ('Divergence').

Before the 1990s: Early developments

Laura's story I: A parent's experience

Laura, the mother of a 43-year-old daughter with Down's Syndrome, said:

"I still remember the moment, just after my labour, when I heard and learned from the dialogue among the medical staff in the delivery room that my daughter had Down's Syndrome; no one came up to me and informed me directly. I felt helpless and did not know where to seek help or get more information. Afterwards, no social worker came to me to give me any support or counselling. The hospital also did not follow up on my situation after we were discharged. I took some time to accept this news, and I had to seek information from other organisations on my own. The days were full of tears, as I recall." (A scenario from the year 1974)

Laura's experience reflects the general situation of families with a child with intellectual disability in the early 1970s. This period marked the beginning of the development of disability services (then conceived of as 'rehabilitation services') in Hong Kong. From the 1970s to the

1990s, the field was in a developmental phase in ideology, policy direction, service provision and people's understanding.

Morninghill School was the first special school in Hong Kong for pupils with intellectual disability. It was established in 1964 by a group of parents. The school had one class, with four pupils: one each from the USA, Canada, Australia and Scotland. From 1968 the school was subsidised by the government and run by the Hong Kong Association for the Mentally Handicapped (now called Hong Chi Association) (Hong Chi Association, 2018). The enactment by the government of six-year compulsory education in 1971 and nine-year free and compulsory education in 1978 (Poon-McBrayer and Lian, 2002) gradually provided children with intellectual disability the opportunity of schooling. For adults, the first sheltered workshop was established by St James' Settlement in 1973 (Kong, 1997), marking the start of formal intellectual disability services. Later, piecemeal services were provided predominantly by charity organisations with missionary purposes, such as St James' Settlement, Caritas and the Society of Homes for Handicapped (currently Fu Hong Society) (Yeung, 2005). The Hong Kong government did not take a more active role until 1977, when it released the first White Paper on rehabilitation, titled 'Integrating the disabled into the community: a united effort'. It attempted to define different disability groups and proposed a service plan to meet the needs of people with disabilities for the upcoming 10 years (Hong Kong Government, 1977). The spectrum of disability services widened, to include day activity centres for adults with moderate to severe intellectual disabilities, vocational centres or sheltered workshops for adults with mild to moderate intellectual disabilities, and residential services.

Story of Wah and her mother, Mrs Wong (I)

Wah was born in 1965 and was assessed as having a moderate intellectual disability when aged six. Mrs Wong had no idea about Wah's condition before the assessment, simply observing that Wah was somewhat different from other children. The family tried to enrol her in kindergarten, but unfortunately she was rejected by different kindergartens.

In 1972, Wah received her first formal education, in a service centre run by the Hong Kong Association for the Mentally Handicapped. According to Mrs Wong, there was no special school for students with intellectual disabilities at that time. In 1974, the service centre became a special school and was subsidised by the government.

Although the school curriculum focused on self-care skills, Wah was able to develop her talents and potential. She received many awards in different inter-school competitions and at age 18 she became the first female representative of Hong Kong to join an international sports event.

Wah was accepted into a sheltered workshop in the late 1980s and worked on packaging.

The 1977 White Paper became the blueprint for rehabilitation services. The quantity of services gradually increased. By 1990, there were 38 special schools with 5,046 places (Chow, 1991). Places in sheltered workshops increased to 3,315 (Kong, 1997). The government had adopted the concept of segregation, and most services were located away from residential areas. The work tasks in sheltered workshops were usually simple and repetitive packaging jobs. People received minimal self-care training, which was neither real-life nor age-appropriate. Staff adopted an authoritarian and controlling approach to 'manage' service users (Wong, 2006). However, from the late 1980s, normalisation began to influence practitioners in Hong Kong (Lee, 1991).

Mrs Wong (II)

After Wah's rejection by kindergartens, Mrs Wong treasured her place in the special school. "At that time, I thought as a parent I should understand what Wah had learned in school and then I could do the same exercises with her at home. Therefore, I asked the school if I could participate in or observe the teaching process."

Mrs Wong advocated for a social worker in schools for students with moderate intellectual disabilities (there was already a social worker in schools for students with mild disabilities). She said, "I convinced other parents of the importance of having a social worker. I voiced this request in a mass meeting where I spoke in front of the public and government representatives. Although I was scared, I knew I did right." By the year of her daughter's graduation, a social worker had been hired in the school.

In 1987, a significant parents' group, The Hong Kong Joint Council of Parents of Mentally Handicapped (HKJCPMH), was formed. Mrs Wong was a founding member.

Laura (II)

Laura said:

> "I knew other parents from other parents' groups. We started to meet more frequently by arranging group physiotherapy training for our children, and gradually we also grouped together and started our own self-help group, called the Intellectually Disabled Education and Advocacy League (IDEAL), in 1989."

As William Chang, pioneer of parent advocacy in Hong Kong and the first chairperson of HKJCPMH, said, under traditional Chinese culture, parents were hesitant to engage and challenge the government officials. They could not imagine that they could fight for the rights of their children (Chang, 1997). Traditional Chinese values viewed intellectual disability as a cause of shame and the fault of the parents (Yeung, 2005). After experiencing loss, confusion and helplessness in the 1970s, in the mid-1980s parents like Laura and Mrs Wong began to speak out for themselves and their children, prompted by a serious shortage of services and widespread social stigma. The government had failed to provide planned services on schedule. It had promised in 1986 to provide 4,270 places in five years but by 1989 could only offer 1,350 places (Chang, 1997). Furthermore, at that time Hong Kong citizens showed strong antipathy towards people with intellectual disabilities. A number of proposed service centres were rejected in different areas (HKJCPMH, nd). For this reason, from the mid-1980s, parent self-help groups were established with two main functions: mutual support and advocacy.

In summary, the release of the 1977 White Paper on rehabilitation was a watershed, committing government to take a more active role rather than depending on religious charities to provide services. Services started in the 1970s and increased quantitatively in the late 1980s. In the 1970s, foreigners living in Hong Kong organised their own services. After official provision of rehabilitation services, local people began to receive formal services. Parents evolved from experiencing a sense of helplessness in the early 1970s to forming advocacy and mutual-help networks in the late 1980s.

1990–99: The Golden Era

The Golden Era represented a significant step in development at all levels. 'Golden' is a relative concept. This era was better than the two periods before or after. The government increased its emphasis on the rights of people with disabilities as citizens and on legal protections. Services improved remarkably in both quantity and quality. Both people with intellectual disabilities and family members began to get involved in advisory bodies.

Mr Lee (I): Witnessing the rapid increase in the quantity of available services

Mr Lee said:

> "My daughter, with a severe grade of intellectual disability, was born in 1998. It was after the release of the White Paper on rehabilitation in 1995, which was described as the golden harvest period for a rehabilitation service plan. Thus, there were many new service units and a great increase in places."

In 1995, a second White Paper, 'Equal opportunities and full participation: a better tomorrow for all', was released. In this policy paper, the government aimed at achieving equal opportunities for and full participation by people with disabilities (Hong Kong Government, 1995). At the legislative level, the Disability Discrimination Ordinance went into full operation in December 1996 and was enforced by the Equal Opportunities Commission. After strong discontent shown by parents' associations because the Mental Health Ordinance (amended in 1988) defined people with intellectual disabilities as persons with a mental disorder (Chang, 1997), and after repeated complaints from service providers that the ordinance failed to provide adequate legal protection for them (Hong Kong Government, 1995), the ordinance (Cap. 136) was amended for the third time in August 1997. That amendment provided clear distinctions between intellectual disability and mental illness. Nevertheless, the ordinance adopted the umbrella term of 'mentally incapacitated', which aroused additional dissatisfaction. One new measure resulting from the amended ordinance was the establishment, in 1999, of the Guardianship Board of Hong Kong, intended to promote the welfare, interests and protection of adults who were 'mentally incapacitated' (Guardianship Board, 2007). However, its establishment was controversial because it was questioned whether adults with intellectual disabilities should be deprived of their rights as adults simply because of their disability.

With regard to the number of services available, the government endorsed many new service projects. The increase in adult services provided in the decade 1990–99 was the most dramatic in history (see Table 1).

Table 1: Number of service places provided for people with intellectual disabilities by the government

Type(s) of service	1990–91[1]	1998–99[2]	2003[3]	2009[4]	2015[5]
Sheltered workshops, supported employment and/or integrated vocational and rehabilitation services	3,875	7,225	9,297	10,443	11,296
Day activity centres	1,473	3,426	3,881	4,442	5,146
Hostel for adults with moderate/ severe intellectual disabilities	1,384	3,487	4,440	5,190	5,945

Sources:
[1] Working Party on Rehabilitation Policies and Services of Hong Kong Government (1992)
[2] Social Welfare Department (1998)
[3] Social Welfare Department (2003)
[4] Social Welfare Department (2009)
[5] Social Welfare Department (2015)

The combined influence of the concept of community integration and the policy direction of the 1995 White Paper stressed participation in society. The concept was manifest in adult services in three ways: the location of service centres, daily service planning and community education. Firstly, the government attempted to open service centres in housing estates or residential regions (Kong, 1996) to achieve geographical integration. Government and rehabilitation agencies had to consult the opinion of local residents before any new services could be located there. Despite this, a large number of service units were built. Secondly, social workers planned services and organised daily activities using the principle of social integration (Wong, 2006). People with intellectual disabilities were encouraged to interact with their neighbours, through shopping or taking a walk. Thirdly, community education programmes were frequently organised with the aim of increasing public awareness and understanding of intellectual disability.

'Skill for Life', published by the Hong Kong Social Welfare Department in 1992, was a training handbook for adults with intellectual disabilities. It included skills in eight domains: motor, self-care, domestic work, communication, community living, social behaviour, and general recreational and vocational domains. This was the dominant approach in adult services in the 1990s (Wong, 2006). It reflected the prevalence of the individual model of disability, which emphasised the enhancement of personal competence to help the individual adapt to social expectations. In the late 1990s, the concept of quality of life (QoL), proposed by Robert Schalock and colleagues, was introduced through a three-year pioneer QoL project organised by St James' Settlement (Wong, 1999). The project was appealing because of its person-centred approach and emphasis on holistic development by means of different-level interventions, instead of fragmented skills training at the personal level.

However, due to a scarcity of land in Hong Kong, a preference for large-scale living-units has long hindered fully actualising person-centred ideologies. Units of between 33 and 100 beds were the formal service arrangement, and 50-bedded units were the most common provision for adults in the 1990s (Wong, 2004). Such collective living arrangements inevitably created challenges for respecting individuals' needs and personal space.

Mrs Wong (III)

In the early 1990s, the operation of the sheltered workshop where Wah was working was transferred from the government to a non-government organisation (NGO). Later on, parents were welcome to visit the workshop to observe the daily work of their children and were invited to participate in service improvement.

During this era, the development of parent associations also peaked in terms of the empowered level of their leaders, the active participation level of the parents, the number of associations formed and the active exchange of ideas among parents from mainland China, Taiwan and Macau.

According to Chang (1997), the major roles of parents' self-help groups at that time were to provide mutual support, monitor services and lobby for implementation of policies. Parents' groups gained positive feedback from the public as well as government. These groups submitted papers, organised petitions, met with legislative councillors, and organised mass meetings to draw greater government and public attention. Meanwhile, in 1993, the Rehabilitation Advisory Committee, which formulated and monitored rehabilitation policies in Hong Kong, decided to nominate a representative from a parents' group to join the committee (Hong Kong Government, 1995). It was a remarkable step for the Hong Kong parent advocacy movement.

People with intellectual disabilities also achieved a breakthrough in advocacy. Inspired by the European and North American people-first and self-advocacy movements in the 1980s, a group of young people formed Chosen Power in 1995, the first People-First in Asia (Chosen Power, nd). Up to 1999, the self-advocates of Chosen Power attended the first and second local Disability Employment Summit and People-First conference/international conferences, organised in the USA, Malaysia and mainland China. Locally, Chosen Power aims to support more people to speak up for themselves and to critically respond to government policies (Chosen Power, nd).

During the Golden Era the mindsets of policy-makers and practitioners were open to change, mirroring the paradigm shift in the international field. The advocacy movement both among people with intellectual disabilities and their family members developed substantially.

Although there was a significant increase in services, in 1999 there were still long waiting lists, and most applicants for residential services had to wait for four to five years (Audit Commission, 1999). A shortage of services has long been the number-one challenge for the government, and that challenge worsened in the twenty-first century.

The Millennium to the present: Divergence

From 2000 onwards, there were unprecedented challenges for families and people with intellectual disabilities. The mechanisms for welfare review and planning established previously were neither continued nor replaced. Families and people with intellectual disabilities continue to be influenced by global trends, and their concerns are no longer restricted to welfare but now also include human rights, self-determination and service diversity.

After 1997 (when Britain transferred sovereignty over Hong Kong to China), the government ceased issuing White Papers, which provided guiding principles and policy direction, in relation to people with a disability. This suspension caused a loss of focus and vision. In contrast to other countries, Hong Kong has never taken proactive legislative steps to formulate policies for people with disabilities (Wong and Wong, 2007). There are no specific Acts in relation to education and employment for people with disabilities in Hong Kong. This has meant a lack of protection for special school and employment provision.

The UN Convention on the Rights of Persons with Disabilities (UNCRPD) has been applicable in Hong Kong since 2008. However, the UNCRPD Civil Committee has commented that the government has done very little to echo the Convention's requirements. For example, the dignity and rights of people with disabilities still have not been adequately protected by the Disability Discrimination Ordinance, the Mental Health Ordinance and the Design Manual (UNCRPD Civil Committee, 2012). The United Nations (2012) has also commented that government has been inadequate in legally protecting people from sexual violence. For example, sexual abuse court cases have been repeatedly suspended because the victims were not fit to be cross-examined (Civil Society Law Reform Committee, 2017).

The government has not committed to developing a community living model. Further, it has failed to speed up the provision of residential homes. In September 2017, there were 4,660 applicants waiting for residential homes (Social Welfare Department, 2017), with the longest waiting time extending more than 17 years. One measure by the government for tackling the terribly long queue is to provide rehabilitation complexes instead. These complexes are multi-storey with many service units where up to a thousand people work and/or live. Ultimately, Hong Kong has never successfully put deinstitutionalisation into practice.

Mr Lee (II)

Mr Lee said:

> "My daughter has had a gastrostomy since one year ago. Her only choice of a living arrangement after special schooling is to go to Siu Lam Hospital (an infirmary). I cannot accept my daughter spending her remaining life in Siu Lam Hospital – the physical setting is that of a traditional hospital. There are more than 300 people in the hospital now, with around 50 people in a ward. People who stay there are called 'patients' and treated as patients; for example, they do not have their own clothes or personal belongings. I don't want her to live as a patient for the rest of her life. I want her to receive more humanistic care, such as having more social and recreational engagement so that she can visit the community and know more about life outside the hospital."

Laura (III)

Laura said:

> "Feeling helpless since the birth of my daughter, I have experienced the obvious service gap in support of families, especially when the needs of my child have overlapped in different government departments in medical, educational, psychological and social aspects. Not a single department follows the cases of people with intellectual disabilities as a family unit or as a lifelong intervention. Services are divided in accord with age, and often neglect the needs of families, too. Therefore, we now advocate for case management."

The experiences of Mr Lee and Laura may reflect the helplessness and limited choices under the current system and practices. The lack of strong coordination across the governmental departments (Wong and Wong, 2007) makes it difficult to fully manifest the principles of a social model. At the service level, a systematic case management approach across different governmental systems and departments is still absent in Hong Kong (Law and Shek, 2016; Lyu and Hui, 2017). This omission causes many families to suffer, and the services they receive are often piecemeal, not tailor-made, inefficient and ineffective.

Wah (IV): Wah's experiences in a sheltered workshop and a hostel

Wah said:

> "I have been in this sheltered workshop* for more than 20 years. The main task is to pack one-off tableware for a fast food chain. The job has never changed up to the present [January 2018]."

Wah moved into a hostel seven years ago. When talking about whether she likes to live in the hostel, she asked immediately, "Why do I need to enter a hostel?" She rated the experience of living in hostel as a 4 on a 10-point scale, whereas she ranked living at home with her mother as a 10. She responded that home is better and quieter.

Note: * The Hong Kong government still uses the term 'sheltered workshop'. It reflects a continued segregated and protective approach in vocational training.

Wah's statement demonstrates that the service model of sheltered workshops has not changed much in the past two decades. Her question 'Why do I need to enter a hostel?' reflects the reality of limited choices for people with intellectual disabilities and their parents. Mrs Wong, in her eighties, understands that she has to leave Wah someday. Because of the lack of community-based services/support in Hong Kong, the only choice for Wah is to live in a hostel after her mother's death.

However, in line with the ideas of quality of life and self-determination, academics and practitioners have attempted to introduce innovative projects. For example, self-determination projects have been carried out with the aim to maximise opportunities for daily choices and decision-making for service users (Wong, 2015). A number of social enterprise projects are run by NGOs, such as restaurants, bakeries and pottery studios, that aim to provide employment opportunities and also help the general public recognise people's work talents.

Whereas the Hong Kong government's mindset about disability is lagging behind the international trend, people with intellectual disabilities and caregivers are moving in the direction of human rights. The signing of the UNCRPD has had a significant impact. For example, in 2012, a member of Chosen Power attended the seventh hearing of the UNCRPD at Geneva. Chosen Power members have also delivered presentations on various issues in the Legislation Council's public hearings (Chosen Power, nd). Parents also understand that their influence has to take place through elections and pressure on the policy-makers to ensure that disability is an agenda item. Mr Lee decided to join the election committee subsector for elections (for electing Hong Kong Special Administrative Region's Chief Executive) in 2016, as the only representative of the intellectual disability field.

Since the Millennium, the government's pace and mindset have seemed to lag behind the global trend. Faced with this, people with intellectual disabilities and their caregivers have adopted a bottom-up approach to influencing government. Their appeals have no longer been confined to the welfare-seeking level but have urged a focus on human rights and the social model of disability.

Conclusion

A review of Hong Kong's 50-year history of providing services for people with intellectual disabilities shows significant developments during the 1990s but only minimal progress in the two decades since. However, inspired by the UNCRPD, people with intellectual disabilities and caregivers seek policy reform emphasising human rights. There are still a number of long-standing challenges, such as a serious shortage of services, along with new challenges, such as a double-ageing issue (both parents and their children). There is an urgent call for the government to adopt a contemporary philosophy that will drive a policy shift to address the changing needs of people with intellectual disabilities and their families.

References

Audit Commission (1999) *Services for students with special educational needs*, Hong Kong: Audit Commission.

Chang, W. (1997) 'Cong jia zhang jiao du kan "fu quan": hui ying she hui fu li shu shu zhang' ['Empowerment from the perspective of a parent: in response to the director of the social welfare department'], in Y.L. Choy and T.W. Yeung (eds) *Xiang gang ruo zhi cheng ren fu wu: hui gu ji zhan wang*, Hong Kong: Chung Hwa Book Co, pp 43–52.

Chosen Power (nd) *Chosen power history*. Available from: http://cppfhk. blogspot.hk/ (accessed 14 December 2017).

Chow, L.Y.H. (1991) 'Jian jie xiang gang ruo zhi er tong jiao yu' ['Introduction of services for children with intellectual disabilities'], in K.M. Ming, K.M. Sham, S.H. Tong, K.M. Hui, and S.Y. Lai (eds), *Shi fen zhen hi fen xin: xiang gang ruo zhi fu wu wen ji*, Hong Kong: Hong Kong Association of Workers Serving the Mentally Handicapped, pp 123–5.

Civil Society Law Reform Committee (2017) *Better protection of legal rights for vulnerable victims/witnesses*, Hong Kong: Civil Society Law Reform Committee.

Guardianship Board (2007) *The 2003–2006 second report*, Hong Kong: Guardianship Board.

HKJCPMH (Hong Kong Joint Council of Parents of the Mentally Handicapped) (nd) *History*. Available from https://www.hkjcpmh. org.hk/zh-hant/history (accessed 18 January 2018).

Hong Chi Association (2018) *History*. Available from: www.hongchi. org.hk/en_about_history.asp (accessed 15 January 2018).

Hong Kong Government (1977) *White Paper on rehabilitation: Integrating the disabled into the community: A united effort*, Hong Kong: Hong Kong Government Printer.

Hong Kong Government (1995) *White Paper on rehabilitation: Equal opportunities and full participation: A better tomorrow for all*, Hong Kong: Hong Kong Government Printer.

Kong, S.K. (1996) 'Social work in the rehabilitation field', in I. Chi and S.K. Cheung (eds), *Social work in Hong Kong*, Hong Kong: Hong Kong Social Workers Association, pp 46–56.

Kong, S.K. (1997) 'Bi hu gong chang de xin tiao zhan' ['New challenges of sheltered workshop'], in Y.L. Choy and T.W. Yeung (eds), *Xiang gang ruo zhi cheng ren fu wu: hui gu ji zhan wang*, Hong Kong: Chung Hwa Book Co, pp 65-80.

Law, B.M. and Shek, D.T.L. (2016) 'Services for people with intellectual and developmental disabilities in Hong Kong', in I.L. Rubin, D.E. Greydanus, J. Merrick and D.R. Patel (eds), *Health care for people with intellectual and developmental disabilities across the lifespan*, Cham, Switzerland: Springer, pp 471-481.

Lee, T.K. (1991) 'Zheng chang hua – kang fu gong zuo zhi yuan ze' ['Normalisation – Principle of rehabilitation work'], in K.M. Ming, K.M. Sham, S.H. Tong, K.M. Hui and S.Y. Lai (eds), *Shi fen zhen, shi fen xin: xiang gang ruo zhi fu wu wen ji*, Hong Kong: Hong Kong Association of Workers Serving the Mentally Handicapped, pp 21–9.

Lyu, Y.F. and Hui, N.N.A. (2017) 'Zhi zhang ren shi ge an guan li de yuan jing: ge an guan li ju li zhen zheng hui ji zhi zhang ren shi hai you duo yuan – xu qiu yu xian zhuang' ['Vision on case management of people with intellectual disability: how far could case management truly be beneficial to people with intellectual disability – needs and current situation'], in Y.C. Yeung (ed), *We care we share*, Hong Kong: The Intellectual Disabled Education and Advocacy League, pp 97–125.

Poon-McBrayer, K.F. and Lian, M.J. (2002) *Special needs education: Children with exceptionalities*, Hong Kong: The Chinese University Press.

Social Welfare Department (1998) *The five-year plan for social welfare development in Hong Kong*, Hong Kong.

Social Welfare Department (2003) *Social Welfare Department Annual Report: Services for People with Disabilities*, Hong Kong.

Social Welfare Department (2009) *Social Welfare Department Annual Report: Services for People with Disabilities*, Hong Kong

Social Welfare Department (2015) *Social Welfare Department Annual Report: Services for People with Disabilities*, Hong Kong.

Social Welfare Department (2017) *Information on number of applications waitlisted in the central referral system for rehabilitation services (Note 1)*, *Hong Kong*. Available from: https://www.swd.gov.hk/storage/asset/section/687/tc/Annex_II_Eng_20170930.pdf

UNCRPD Civil Committee (2012) *Hong Kong shadow report on United Nations Convention on the Rights of Persons with Disabilities*, Hong Kong: Civil Committee.

United Nations (2012) *Concluding observations on the initial report of China, adopted by the Committee at its eighth session*, Geneva: The United Nations.

Wong, P.K.S. (1999) 'Actualize the quality of life concept: a way to change the lives of people with intellectual disabilities', in *Newsletter*, vol 12, Hong Kong: Hong Kong Joint Council of Parents of the Mentally Handicapped.

Wong, P.K.S. (2004) *Evaluating a staff development programme using an interpersonal-environment approach to facilitating self-determination of adults with intellectual disabilities in Hong Kong: A pretest–posttest control group design*, unpublished MPhi. thesis, Hong Kong: The University of Hong Kong.

Wong, P.K.S (2006) 'Zhi zhang ren shi ri jian fu wu de yan bian ji qu shi' ['The trend of day services for adults with intellectual disabilities'], *Ge ren, jia ting, she qu fu kang fu wu zheng he xin ti yan*, Hong Kong: Salvation Army, pp 35–49.

Wong, P.K.S. (2015) *Relational and contextual self-determination: Qualitative and quantitative studies of adults with mild intellectual disability in Hong Kong*, unpublished PhD thesis, Hong Kong: The University of Hong Kong.

Wong, P.K.S. and Wong, D.F.K. (2007) 'Disability', in *Consultancy team, envisioning social welfare: Our shared future*. Hong Kong: Department of Social Work and Social Administration, The University of Hong Kong, pp 96–110.

Working Party on Rehabilitation Policies and Services of Hong Kong Government (1992) *Green Paper on equal opportunities and full participation: A better tomorrow for all*, Hong Kong.

Yeung, Y.C. (2005) 'A narrative analysis of fathers' experiences having a child with intellectual disability', unpublished PhD thesis, Hong Kong: Chinese University of Hong Kong.

SEVEN

People with intellectual disabilities in the European semi-periphery: the case of Hungary

Ágnes Turnpenny

Introduction

This chapter gives an overview of the changing situation of people with intellectual disabilities throughout the twentieth century in Hungary. The analysis follows four broad historical periods: before the end of the Second World War; state socialism between 1945 and 1989; the period of post-socialist transformation from 1990; and the current period following Hungary's European Union membership in 2004. Although these periods were far from homogenous from a socio-political perspective, nevertheless taking a broad chronological approach helps to highlight and trace change and continuity in the situation of people with intellectual disabilities across the decades.

The chapter primarily draws on historical sources as well as the analysis of published data and research, and also includes three vignettes constructed to illustrate some 'typical themes' in the life trajectories of individuals with intellectual disabilities and their families in contemporary Hungary, highlighting the various forms of exclusion they face. The vignettes are based on themes emerging from real-life stories and quantitative quality-of-life research; however, they do not relate to any specific individuals. Any similarities to real-life stories are coincidental.

Before 1945

In Hungary until the Second World War the family and the local community (municipality) were the main providers of care to people with intellectual disabilities. The first institution and residential school for children with intellectual disabilities opened in the capital, Budapest, in 1875. This was followed by the establishment of several special (remedial) classes and 'orthopedagogic institutions' across the country.

The Population Census of 1881 identified 18,672 individuals with intellectual disabilities,[1] a rate of 12 per 10,000 population (Országos Magyar Királyi Statisztikai Hivatal [National Royal Statistical Office], 1882, 776). According to Jakab Frim, the founder of the first institution, the treatment of people with intellectual disabilities in Hungary at the time was comparable to countries 'we do not like to be compared with' and was lagging far behind 'modern Western countries' (1884, 94). He described the situation of people with intellectual disabilities in bleak terms: '[o]ften families keep them hidden in the house, sometimes they are abandoned, or placed with families or in charitable hospitals at the lowest possible cost' (Frim, 1884, 81). Local authorities issued begging licences to those who were not supported by their families; thus, the majority of adults with disabilities lived in 'extreme and shocking poverty' (Kemény, 1888).

Orthopedagogy and special education for children with learning difficulties and sensory impairments were established in Hungary based on Austrian and German models in the early twentieth century. This contrasted with a complete lack of support and services for children and adults with more severe intellectual disabilities. Mortality, especially infant mortality, was very high compared to Western Europe (Tomka, 2002) and the killing of disabled, terminally ill or frail elderly people was practised in some rural communities until the Second World War (Horváth, 1988).

Begging was prohibited in 1936 and municipalities were called to strengthen provision for vulnerable groups; however, this did not happen. Authorities and the community failed to acknowledge the importance of adequate provision for people with disabilities (Schuler, 1937). The first charitable association for adults with intellectual disabilities[2] was established in 1930 and one of its aims was to create a network of residential institutions across the country. The association set up a campus for adults with intellectual disabilities in Budapest and opened another home in nearby Dunakeszi. Some adults with intellectual disabilities were placed in psychiatric hospitals or 'family care colonies'. Conditions in psychiatric hospitals were extremely poor and mortality associated with malnutrition and tuberculosis was high (Baran and Gazdag, 2006).

The first half of the twentieth century saw the rise of eugenic ideas about the social and biological control of the population. In the words of Mitchell and Snyder (2003), 'as one of the first truly trans-Atlantic scientific movements, eugenics bound much of Europe, the United

States and Canada in a concerted movement to rid disabilities from their own national spaces' (p 856). Although eugenics was a popular ideology in Hungary and had many proponents across the political spectrum, the agendas pursued arose from local conditions and realities, in particular the territorial and political changes following the Peace Treaty of Trianon in 1920, and thus were most closely interlinked with the nation state, racial nationalism and national renewal (Turda and Weindling, 2006, 7). In this context the primary concern of eugenic policies was the 'preservation of the Hungarian race' against minorities, in particular Jews and to a lesser extent the Roma, also promoting pronatalist family and public health measures (Turda, 2013; Varsa 2017a). Even though the eugenic sterilisation of people with certain disabilities and congenital conditions was advocated by some and even debated in the Hungarian Parliament in the 1930s, this was never adopted (Turda and Weidling, 2006, 8).

The Second World War left the country devastated with over a million casualties, including nearly 500,000 Jews and over 10,000 Roma murdered in the Holocaust (Stark, 1989, 1995; Braham, 2000; Bársony and Daróczi, 2008). Unlike in Austria or Germany, in Hungary there were no systematic attempts to exterminate people with intellectual disabilities (Mitchell and Snyder, 2003). Nevertheless, the war most likely had a catastrophic effect on the lives of vulnerable individuals, especially those living in long-stay hospitals, many of whom died due to starvation, poor hygiene and epidemics (Baran and Gazdag, 2006).

Between 1948 and 1989: the years of state socialism

After the war, the new, democratically elected government planned to introduce a social-democratic welfare model. Social policy became government responsibility (as opposed to municipal responsibility before the war) and the Ministry of Social Welfare was established. However, this period was short-lived and following the transition to Communism (and erosion of post-war democratic institutions) between 1946 and 1949, the development of social policy took a new direction (Kenez, 2006; Romsics, 2010, ch IV.2). In the words of Szalai and Orosz (1992):

> [T]he new system abolished social policy in general. All of its traditional institutions were cast away as the requisites of overthrown capitalism. At the same time – and it was the essence of its self-contradiction – the 'socialist'

planned economy was regarded as the main trustee of social rationality and the social good. It followed that each and every segment of economy and society, of private and public life, became imbued with 'social' considerations as the central intention. (p 149)

The 'socialist' welfare state was organised around the principle of full employment. All adults – men and women – were required to work except those who were considered too frail or too disabled. Those who did not want to work were labelled as 'workshy', which also became a criminal category and could mean imprisonment or institutionalisation (Szikra and Tomka, 2009).

Children with disabilities were seen as a hindrance to their families. Parents who did not want to send their children to institutions and decided to look after them at home received no support from the state. This was also strongly disapproved by professionals (eg paediatricians) and the general public; until relatively recently women were often encouraged to abandon disabled newborn babies in maternity wards (Bass, 2004; Kálmán, 2004). Children with more severe disabilities were labelled 'ineducable' and excluded from public education until 1993.

The expansion of residential care for children – children's homes and child protection institutions – was also used as a means both to enable and to enforce women's entry into paid employment. Prejudice against Romani mothers as 'workshy' was prevalent in child protection and resulted in the institutionalisation of many children (Varsa, 2009; Varsa, 2017b). Romani children would be disproportionately labelled as having 'intellectual disabilities' and institutionalised for life (ERRC, 2007; Kende and Neményi, 2006).

M's story

M is 42 years old and lives in an institution in a small village in a deprived area of Hungary. The nearest town is a 20-minute drive away but public transport is infrequent and expensive.

The institution was established in the 1980s and currently accommodates over 150 people with intellectual disabilities. The majority need little support with activities of daily living. The institution has sheltered workshops and a large vegetable allotment on site where many of the residents work. Most people have no or limited contact with their families and many come from disadvantaged Roma backgrounds.

M had a difficult childhood: she was removed from her family at the age of five by social services due to the chaotic family environment and grew up in a children's home. She lost contact with her family, although she is aware that her parents passed away and some of her siblings also live in a social care institution.

M has learning difficulties and finished her compulsory education in a special needs primary school. She left school aged 16 with no qualifications. She moved to the institution aged 19 from the children's home and has lived here since. She works as a cleaner in the institution 15 hours a week and gets paid below the minimum wage. She shares a room with two other women. They are proud of their room for which they picked the colour, curtains and rugs. She has a long-term partner who also lives in the institution.

M feels settled, has some friends and goes on annual holidays organised by the institution. She dislikes the noise and the lack of privacy; she would love to have her own bathroom and more independence.

The institution is currently undergoing transformation: residents will move into supported housing with eight to 12 places in the village and surrounding areas. There was some initial resistance from the community – fearing that crime and antisocial behaviour would increase in the village if residents "could live and go out freely" – but the move is finally going ahead.

M is expected to move into a house with seven others and will share a room with her partner. M is looking forward to the move, especially the better living conditions, more freedom and opportunities to do things that she enjoys, such as cooking. But even after the move, they will eat lunch in the institution canteen each day.

M and her partner would also like to get married but as they are both under guardianship, this has not been possible.

At the same time, residential institutions were seen as an opportunity to create employment for large numbers of unskilled (mostly female) workers in rural areas not reached by large-scale industrialisation. New institutions were established in a huge variety of nationalised buildings – mansion houses, convents, warehouses, army barracks and so on – located on the outskirts of villages or in remote areas, often close to the country's western and eastern borders (Horváth, 1988; Ficsorné, 2009).

Even though social care was the responsibility of the Ministry of Health from 1950, residential institutions were not formally part of the health-care system and were chronically underfunded. Residential institutions resembled the old charitable hospitals and accommodated mixed groups of people who were unable or unwilling to work, including people with disabilities, elderly people, people with mental health problems, those with substance abuse problems, anti-social behaviour or even certain long-term health conditions, primarily tuberculosis. Physical conditions were extremely poor; inadequate hygiene facilities, overcrowding and the lack of personal space were common features (Horváth, 1988).

There were some early attempts to create separate institutions for people with intellectual disabilities with the establishment of some work-based institutions (in Hungarian: *foglalkoztató intézet*) in the mid-1950s. These were primarily for young adults with mental health problems but some accommodated people with intellectual disabilities (Benedek, 1957). They were typically located close to large collective farms and provided residents with seasonal agricultural and light industrial work.

When Western countries started to embark on deinstitutionalisation in the 1970s, Hungary set out to consolidate institutional care for people with disabilities. New legislation distinguished two types of institutions: work-based institutions (later known as 'rehabilitation institutions') and social care homes, and the 'profile-cleaning' of existing institutions got under way. This meant the reallocation of residents between settings on the basis of their disability and needs to create specialist provision.

The impact on people's everyday lives was significant: people were moved often without any consultation or preparation: for example, they found out in the morning that they would be moving to a new institution in the afternoon. Horváth (1988) suggests that it 'is impossible to know how many people had to move as a result of profile cleaning and thus how many people lost their social contacts or moved to a new environment' (p 58).

At the same time there was also a substantial expansion of capacity and new institutions were established. Between 1970 and 1990 the number of places in institutions for people with intellectual disabilities nearly tripled from 3,200 to 10,600 (Népjóléti Minisztérium [Ministry of Welfare], 1990). Some of these were in new, purpose-built settings, but the majority occupied existing buildings, such as the institution in Darvastó that was established in 1983 on an abandoned bauxite mining site to accommodate people with 'mild and moderate' intellectual disabilities from Budapest, nearly 200 kilometres from the city. Thus, living conditions did not improve significantly during this period. The government's plan was that 10% of the total population with 'mild' and 70% of people with 'moderate' intellectual disabilities would be looked after in work-based institutions and all people with severe and profound intellectual disabilities would have a place in social care homes (Hermányi, 1985).

The first non-residential services for people with intellectual disabilities were established in the 1970s: these included sheltered workshops and day care centres (Ficsorné, 2009). By the mid-1970s maternity benefits were available for women to stay at home with their children, including children with disabilities (Szikra and Tomka, 2009). This offered an alternative to institutionalisation for many families, although their situation was extremely difficult in the absence of services and support.

Parents started to come together and organise on an informal basis from the 1960s. However, attempts to establish the first association to represent people with intellectual disabilities and their families faced the disapproval of the ruling Socialist Workers' Party (they were the only political party and they controlled the executive power and the Parliament as well) (Ficsorné, 2009).

As the regime softened – in this period was Hungary was often referred to as the 'happiest barrack' – and awareness of disability issues increased, the Committee of Interest Protection of Parents of Intellectually Disabled[3] was eventually established in 1981, the United Nations International Year of Disabled Persons (Baár, 2015). Initially the Committee was part of the Hungarian Association of the Deaf and Hard of Hearing[4] but the organisation became independent and changed its name to the Hungarian Association for Persons with Intellectual Disability (ÉFOÉSZ) in 1989.[5] In the meantime a national network of grass-roots organisations was created – mostly by parents, with the support of some professionals – providing advocacy, peer support and organised cultural and leisure activities for people living with their families. The organisation also had contacts with international partners, primarily its counterpart *Lebenshilfe* in Austria and Germany, who provided much more than just financial support (Ficsorné, 2009, 42).

The idea of deinstitutionalisation first appeared in Hungary in the 1980s among professionals and parents of people with intellectual disabilities who had visited or heard about Austrian, Canadian and US services through these international connections (Lányi-Engelmayer, 1982).

The first group homes opened in the late 1980s, shortly before the fall of the Iron Curtain in 1989. By this time the erosion of the regime had reached a point where private initiatives were no longer prohibited but actively tolerated. This period was also characterised by an intense search for new approaches and openness to new ideas.

ÉFOÉSZ and other grass-roots parent groups increasingly openly voiced concerns over poor conditions and human rights abuses in residential institutions and the lack of community-based alternatives. They advocated community-based services based on Western models. There were also reform attempts in some institutions initiated by open-minded management and individuals with intellectual disabilities seeking more independent living opportunities. These included group homes, 'half-way houses' and even supported living-type arrangements.

P's story

P is 35 years old, has Down's Syndrome and lives with his mother in Budapest, where he also has a married older sister. Their father left the family when P was young; their mother brought up the children with support from her parents, who passed away a few years ago.

P attended special needs primary school and college, and after leaving school started at a day centre three days a week. He needs support using public transport, so his mother accompanies him to and from the centre. However, this is getting increasingly difficult as she is getting older and has health problems herself.

P enjoys the day centre: he has friends and they do different activities, such as arts and crafts and play games. He also loves spending time with his sister's family. He has no other friends and spends most of his free time at home with his mother, usually watching television. Money is extremely tight and they have not been on a holiday together for over 15 years.

His mother is extremely worried about the future when she can no longer look after him. She does not want to 'burden' her daughter but she does not want to send P to an institution either. She would like him to move to a 'family-like' group home but those services are extremely scarce and she cannot afford the one-off payment they often require.

The years of post-socialist transformation: 1990–2004

There seemed to be a prospect of real policy change in the early 1990s amid the increasingly difficult economic situation and fundamental welfare reforms. These reforms were characterised by a decentralisation of social provision, both services and benefits, to municipalities, incorporating a strong element of discretion while failing to provide adequate financial resources. Appeals to the emerging voluntary sector – mostly grass-roots initiatives with limited resources – to fill in gaps in social services were made without the provision of adequate legal framework and funding (Deacon, 2000).

A new law on social care and benefits came into force in 1993 (Act III of 1993) that represented a major departure from the welfare policies of the previous regime in many areas by introducing new measures to tackle the challenges of economic transformation such as long-term unemployment and poverty; however, social care services were left unchanged. The Act preserved the existing system with institutions as the only form of residential service provision for individuals with an intellectual disability. The new legislation failed to take account of already existing community-based services and deinstitutionalisation initiatives. Day services were delegated to municipalities with a population size of 10,000 or more inhabitants, meaning that large numbers of those living in smaller settlements were left without access to any support.

In 1998 the Hungarian Parliament adopted a law on the rights and equal opportunities of people with disabilities (Act XXVI of 1998), which declared that:

> residential institutions for people with disabilities should gradually, but latest by January 1, 2010 be transformed in a way that allows those who are capable of independent living with adequate personal support to live in small-scale group homes, and for those people with severe disabilities who need more intensive support provide humanised and modernised institutional care. (Article 29:5)

Group homes were defined as 'a small-scale residential setting that supports independent living of individuals with disabilities' (Article 4/e). Although some saw this as a mandate for deinstitutionalisation, it turned out not to be the case.

In 1996 the Hungarian Soros Foundation launched a programme entitled *Kitagolás* (outplacement) that aimed to bring out people from institutions to live in group homes in the community, set up according to the principles of normalisation. The programme promoted the adoption of existing models by supporting study visits to Austria, the dissemination of international experiences, as well as the translation of international literature (Kedl, 2002). The annual conferences between 1997 and 2001 brought together government policy-makers and state and voluntary sector service providers, and in the last two years people with intellectual disabilities and their families as well. The perception of the Foundation as an organisation with no vested interest in service provision and its moderate stance on deinstitutionalisation facilitated communication and the acceptance of new ideas.

The other major initiative[6] came from the Dutch government between 1997 and 2002. Independent non-profit organisations – mostly grass-roots parent groups – were supported to set up community-based homes for adults with intellectual disabilities. The project included study visits, staff exchange with Dutch organisations and training programmes. The programme publicity and project successes helped to demonstrate the feasibility of community living to policy-makers and secured some funding for capital investment from the Ministry of Social Affairs.

Although these programmes were instrumental in making community-based group homes an accepted part of social care, they had limitations. Firstly, they did not explicitly challenge the prevailing consensus that saw institutions as an essential part of disability services. Furthermore, by introducing and disseminating the ideas of normalisation and independent living, their vocabulary was incorporated into the very rhetoric of reform and modernisation and helped to preserve institutional care and practices. While rhetorically committed to deinstitutionalisation, the government also continued to fund the refurbishment and expansion of existing institutions via regional development funds directly channelled to local government until the mid-2000s.

In 1999 the Act on Social Care was amended to incorporate 'group homes' as a new form of residential care (alongside institutions). The definition of group homes was very narrow and rigid: a minimum of eight and a maximum of 14 places, for people with low or moderate support needs aged 16–60 years with their own income. These restrictions affected some existing services supporting people with complex needs or with fewer than eight places. Thus, the Act was amended again to replace the single definition of group homes with two new categories that mirrored those of institutions: care group homes and rehabilitation group homes. Although this did not solve the issue of minimum numbers, people with severe disabilities and complex needs could remain in group homes. It also signalled the 'institutionalisation' of community-based services.

Current situation

Hungary joined the European Union in 2004 and unprecedented amounts of money became available for human development, including education, employment and social services. However, policies were set according to EU rules and priorities. Between 2004 and 2006 this was primarily the development of employment opportunities and services for people with disabilities. In 2006 the EU permitted the use of the European Regional Development Fund for investments in 'social infrastructure which contribute to regional and local development and increasing the quality of life' in the new Member States (EC, 2006, Article 4.11).

A's story

A is in his mid-thirties, has autism and learning difficulties. He lives in a group home with nine other people in a town. The service is run by a charity originally established by parents in the mid-1990s. The house was built with grant funding and donations and the charity also established a sheltered workshop, where most of the residents work. Through programmes supported by European structural and investment funds the charity has recently expanded its employment and day services.

A works in the sheltered workshop five days a week and attends regular, scheduled activities with the service including swimming and horse riding. They also go on trips and holidays together. He gets on well with housemates and staff; however, he has no friends outside the home. In the evenings they eat dinner and watch television or play board games together.

A has a close relationship with his family, especially his mother who is very much involved in A's life: she is also his guardian.

In 2007 Hungary was one of the first countries in the world to ratify the UN Convention on the Rights of Persons with Disabilities (CRPD) and its Optional Protocol. This was hailed as an 'outstanding achievement of disability policy' by the government but in reality it paid no more than lip service to disability rights without any consideration of future implementation of the ratification process. Nevertheless, the CRPD was successfully used by disabled people's and human rights organisations to prevent the government's attempt to use EU funds to refurbish institutions and to lobby for the launch of an institutional closure programme in 2012. This programme is still ongoing, but has thus far delivered few tangible results for people with intellectual disabilities living in institutions, and even fewer for those living in the community independently or with their families.

Some old practices which curtail rather than enhance rights have survived, in particular guardianship, which affects a large number of people with intellectual disabilities and represents a major obstacle to community living and inclusion (HCLU, 2015).

By 2017 six institutions – four accommodating people with intellectual disabilities and two for people with psychosocial disabilities – were replaced by smaller homes, primarily group homes for eight to 12 people, close to the site of the institutions. However, not all residents could move to these new settings: out of 770 new places planned only 672 were actually created and many people labelled as 'too disabled' were transferred to other institutions, mostly nursing homes for elderly people (Kozma et al, 2016, 75).

Meanwhile there are still at least 120 institutions for people with intellectual disabilities where more than 14,000 people are excluded from society; it is estimated that one in three people with intellectual disabilities and one in ten autistic people live in an institutional setting (KSH, 2016, Kopasz et al, 2016).

People who live with their families – the majority – also experience high levels of social exclusion and deprivation. Research in the early twenty-first century has shown that people living in the community had limited access to services and support, and were likely to experience poverty (Kopasz et al, 2006; Bernát and Kozma, 2017).

Conclusion

This chapter has highlighted how the situation of people with intellectual disabilities changed in Hungary across the twentieth century. Although during this time the country underwent major political and societal transformation, the exclusion of people with intellectual disabilities – and their families – is a constant feature across historical periods and political regimes. It also seems that Hungary – in the words of Böröcz (2012) – is 'catching up, forever' trying to improve the situation of people with intellectual disabilities by emulating developments in Western countries. However, inertia is strong, and reforms have had limited success so far.

Notes

[1] The term used at the time was '*hülye*' ('stupid' in English), nowadays considered derogatory and used in colloquial language.

[2] In Hungarian: *Szellemileg Elmaradottakat Gyámolító Emberbarátok Országos Egyesülete*.

[3] In Hungarian: *Értelmi Fogyatékosok Szüleinek Országos Érdekvédelmi Szekciója*.

[4] In Hungarian: *Siketek és Nagyothallók Országos Szövetsége*.

[5] In Hungarian: *Értelmi Fogyatékossággal Élők és Segítőik Országos Érdekvédelmi Szövetsége*.

[6] Fészek (Nest) Programme.

References

Baár, M. (2015) 'Informal networks, international developments and the founding of the first interest-representing associations of disabled people in Hungary in the late socialist period (1970s–1980s)', *Moving the Social*, 53, 39–62.

Baran, B., and Gazdag, G. (2006) 'The fate of the Hungarian psychiatric patients during World War II', *International Journal of Mental Health*, 35(4), 88–99.

Bársony, J. and Daróczi, Á. (eds) (2008) *Pharrajimos: The fate of the Roma during the Holocaust*, New York: IDEA.

Bass, L. (2004) 'Szüljön másikat?!' ['Have another one?!'], in L. Bass (ed), *Jelentés a súlyosan-halmozottan fogyatékos embereket nevelő család életkörülményeiről* [*Report on the situation of families caring for people with profound and multiple intellectual disabilities*], Budapest: Kézenfogva Alapítvány, pp 54–91.

Benedek, I. (1957) *Aranyketrec: egy elmeosztály élete* [*Golden cage: Life in a mental ward*], Budapest: Bibliotheca Kiadó.

Bernát, A., and Kozma, Á. (2017) *A fogyatékos nappali ellátásban biztosított fejlesztések, programok, tevékenységek feltáró vizsgálata* [*An exploratory study of day care provision for people with intellectual disabilities in Hungary*], Budapest: TÁRKI (full text in Hungarian at: http://www.tarki.hu/hu/news/2017/kitekint/20170424_nappaliellatas.pdf).

Böröcz, J. (2012) 'Hungary in the European Union: catching up, forever', *Economic & Political Weekly*. XLVIL(22) (9 June).

Braham, R.L. (2000) *The politics of genocide: The Holocaust in Hungary*, Detroit, MI: Wayne State University Press.

Deacon, B. (2000) 'Eastern European welfare states: The impact of the politics of globalization', *Journal of European Social Policy*, 10(2), 146–61.

EC (2006) *Regulation (EC) No 1080/2006 of the European Parliament and of the Council of 5 July 2006 on the European Regional Development Fund and repealing Regulation (EC) No 1783/1999.* Available at: https:// eur-lex.europa.eu/eli/reg/2006/1080/oj

ERRC (European Roma Rights Centre) (2007) *Dis-interest of the child: Romani children in the Hungarian child protection system*, Budapest: ERRC.

Ficsorné, M.K. (2009) 'Az intellektualis fogyatékossággal élő emberek mozgalmának hazai története' ['The history of the advocacy movement of people with intellectual disabilities'], in L. Hegedűs et al (eds) *A fogyatékosügy hazai és nemzetközi története* [*The Hungarian and international history of disabled people's movements*], Budapest, pp 34–66.

Frim, J. (1884) *A hülyeség és a hülyeintézetek, különös tekintettel Magyarország hülyéire* [*Stupidity and institutions for the stupid, with particular attention to Hungary*], Budapest: Posner.

HCLU (Hungarian Civil Liberties Union) (2015) *Sentenced to legal death: People with disabilities can be stripped of their right to decide in Hungary*, Budapest: Hungarian Civil Liberties Union. Available at: https:// tasz.hu/files/tasz/imce/2015/sentenced_to_legal_death_rev_1.pdf

Hermányi, P. (1985) 'Tájékoztatás fontosabb rendeletekről és fejlesztési elképzelésekről' ['Information about key legislation and development plans'], *Szociálpolitikai Értesítő* [*Social Policy Report*], 2.

Horváth, Á. (1988) *A szociális otthon* [*The social care home*], Budapest: MTA Szociológiai Kutató Intézete [HAS Institute for Sociology].

Kálmán, Z. (2004) *Bánatkő. sérült gyermek a családban* [*Grief stone: Disabled child in the family*], Budapest: Bliss Alapítvány.

Kedl, M. (2002) 'A Soros Alapítvány Kitagolás programjának hat éve' ['Six years of the Soros Foundation's Outplacement programme'], in Á. Lányi-Engelmayer (ed) *Kiscsoportos lakóotthonok. hol is tartunk?* [*Small group homes: Where are we now?*], Budapest: Soros Alapítvány, pp 11–20.

Kemény, S. (1888) *Az első magyar hülyék nevelő és ápoló intézetének rövid története* [*Brief history of the first Hungarian institutions of the stupid*], Budapest.

Kende, A. and Neményi, M. (2006) 'Selection in education: the case of Roma children in Hungary', *Equal Opportunities International*, 25(7), 506–22.

Kenez, P. (2006) *Hungary from the Nazis to the Soviets: The establishment of the Communist regime in Hungary, 1944–1948*, Cambridge University Press.

Kopasz, M., Bernát, A., Kozma, Á. and Simonovits, B. (2016) 'Fogyatékossággal élő emberek életminősége Magyarországon az intézménytelenítési folyamat küszöbén' ['The quality of life of people with disabilities in Hungary at the early stages of the deinstitutionalisation process'] in T. Kolosi and Gy. Tóth István (eds) *Társadalmi Riport 2016* [*Social Report 2016*], Budapest: TÁRKI, pp 376–93 (English summary at: http://www.tarki.hu/en/news/2016/items/20160408_fszk_en.pdf).

Kozma, Á., Petri, G., Balogh, A. and Birtha, M. (2016) *Az Európai Unió támogatásainak a szerepe az intézménytelenítésben és a férőhelykiváltás eddigi tapasztalatai* [*The role of EU funding in deinstitutionalisation in Hungary and the experiences of the DI programme so far*], Budapest: Hungarian Civil Liberties Union (English summary at: http://m.cdn.blog.hu/at/ataszjelenti/file/zarotanulmany_tasz_a4_preview_3.pdf).

KSH (2016) *Yearbook of Welfare Statistics 2015*, Budapest: Központi Statisztikai Hivatal (Hungarian Central Statistical Office).

Lányi-Engelmayer, Á. (1982) 'A fogyatékosok szocializációjának lehetséges útjai' ['Possible trajectories for the socialisation of disabled people'], *Gyógypedagógiai Szemle*, 10(4), 279–85.

Mitchell, D., and Snyder, S. (2003) 'The eugenic Atlantic: race, disability, and the making of an international eugenic science, 1800–1945', *Disability & Society*, 18(7), 843–64.

Népjóléti Minisztérium (1990) *Felnőttvédelmi szociális gondoskodás [Adult protection social services]*, Budapest: Népjóléti Minisztérium (Ministry of Social Welfare).

Országos Magyar Királyi Statisztikai Hivatal (1882) *Az 1881. év elején végrehajtott népszámlálás eredményei némely hasznos házi állatok kimutatásával együtt* [*The results of the population census from 1881*], Budapest: Országos Magyar Királyi Statisztikai Hivatal. Available at: https://library.hungaricana.hu/hu/view/NEDA_1881_01/?pg=809&layout=s

Romsics, I. (2011). *Magyarország története a XX. Században [The history of Hungary in the twentieth century]*, Budapest: Osiris. Available at: https://www.tankonyvtar.hu/hu/tartalom/tamop425/2011_0001_520_magyarorszag_tortenete/ch04s02.html

Schuler, D. (1937) *Hatósági és társadalmi embervédelem Budapesten* [*Magisterial and community social protection in Budapest*], Budapest: Budapest Székesfőváros Statisztikai Hivatala (Statistical Office of Budapest Capital City).

Stark, T (1989) *Magyarország második világháborús embervesztesége* [*Casualties of the Second World War in Hungary*], Budapest: MTA TTI.

Stark, T (1995) *Zsidóság a vészkorszakban és a felszabadulás után* [*Jewish people during the Holocaust and after liberation*], Budapest: MTA TTI.

Szalai, J. and Orosz, E. (1992) 'Social policy in Hungary', in B. Deacon (ed), *The new Eastern Europe: Social policy past, present and future*, London: Sage, pp 144–67.

Szikra, D. and Tomka, B. (2009) 'Social policy in East Central Europe: major trends in the 20th century', *Welfare state transformations and adaptations in Central and Eastern Europe*, Palgrave Macmillan: Basingstoke.

Tomka, B. (2002) 'Demographic diversity and convergence in Europe, 1918–1990: the Hungarian case', *Demographic Research*, 6(2), 17–48.

Turda, M. (2013) 'In pursuit of Greater Hungary: eugenic ideas of social and biological improvement, 1940–1941', *The Journal of Modern History*, 85(3), 558–91.

Turda, M. and Weindling, P. (eds) (2007) *'Blood and homeland': Eugenics and racial nationalism in Central and Southeast Europe, 1900–1940*, Budapest: Central European University Press.

Varsa, E (2009) 'Child protection, residential care and the "gypsy-question" in early state socialist Hungary', in S. Hering (ed) *Social care under state socialism (1945–1989)*, Opladen and Farmington Hills: Barbara Budrich Publishers, pp 149–59.

Varsa, E. (2017a) '"The (final) solution of the Gypsy-question": continuities in discourses about Roma in Hungary, 1940s–1950s', *Nationalities Papers*, 45(1), 114–30.

Varsa, E. (2017b) '"The minor would hinder the mother in finding employment": child protection and women's paid work in early state socialist Hungary', *East European Politics and Societies*, 31(4), 818–39.

EIGHT

People with intellectual disabilities in Iceland in the twentieth century: sterilisation, social role valorisation and 'normal life'

Guðrún Stefánsdóttir

Introduction: the Icelandic context

This chapter considers the history of people with intellectual disabilities in Iceland, paying particular attention to the last quarter of the twentieth century when ideas about a normal life began to influence Icelandic disability policy and legislation which has emphasised social equality and participation for over 30 years.

This history is largely a story of discrimination and social exclusion, portraying people with intellectual disabilities as abnormal and inferior. The first half of the twentieth century can be characterised by negative societal views and isolation at institutions. The eugenic movement and the medical understanding of intellectual disabilities played a crucial role in constructing negative societal views of people with intellectual disabilities (Kevles, 1986; Atkinson and Walmsley, 1999). The eugenic movement argued that 'feeble-mindedness' was hereditary and that 'mental defectives' were a threat to society due to their uncontollable urges and degenerative characteristics. The 'professional community', armed with scientific data from hereditary studies, pursued aggressively restrictive measures such as 'controlled marriage, sterilization and segregation through institutionalization' (Scheerenberger, 1983: 154). During the 1920s and 1930s, compulsory sterilisation of women with intellectual disabilities was legalised in many European countries as well as in North America. Such legislation remained in place in most countries until the 1970s and 1980s. This led to involuntary sterilisation of women with intellectual disabilities in many countries (Tilley et al, 2012).

The first Act concerning institutions in Iceland, the Law on Sanctuaries, was passed in 1936 (Alþingi no. 18/1936). This defined the legal framework for the first Icelandic institution. Although the policy was intended to improve people's living conditions it heralded the beginning of institutionalisation in Iceland. Two years later, in 1938, a law was passed legalising sterilisation and abortion for people labelled 'feeble-minded' or with 'another serious disease'. This legislation reflected the influence of eugenics and remained in force until 1975. It was common practice to sterilise women with intellectual disabilities (Karlsdóttir, 1998). In the 1950s, institutions for people with intellectual disabilities came under increasing criticism. Research and official investigations uncovered abusive and dehumanising conditions (Chapman et al, 2015).

During the 1960s and 1970s the ideology of normalisation replaced ideas of segregation and institutionalisation, calling for a 'normal life' for people with intellectual disabilities and advocating for their right to take part in regular community life.

Normalisation ideas reached Iceland at the beginning of the 1970s but it was not until 1979 that the 1936 legislation which set up institutions was revoked. The new legislation reflected the spirit of normalisation and stated the right for people with intellectual disabilities to live an ordinary life and participate in society (Alþingi no. 47/1979). Several years earlier, in 1975, the National Parents Organisation in Iceland had established the first group home in Akureyri and in the capital Reykjavík a year later, in 1976. A new law on services for disabled people in Iceland was enacted in 1992, the Act on the Affairs of Disabled People (Alþingi no. 59/1992). These laws remained in force at the time of writing (2018), with some amendments in 2010, reiterating the obligation to uphold the aims of the Convention on the Rights of People with Disabilities (CRPD). The legislative framework still relies on normalisation, as first established in 1979.

In the early twenty-first century most people with intellectual disabilities live in group homes or in flats located in small apartment buildings. Research demonstrated that people still faced complex barriers in accessing mainstream society and experienced discrimination and prejudice (Stefánsdóttir et al, 2018). With this in mind, it is important to recognise that Iceland ratified the CRPD in 2016 and was, at the time of writing, in the process of finalising draft legislation to bring Icelandic law into alignment with the Convention. The Convention specifically recognises the fulfilment of human rights and the right for persons with disabilities to take an active part in society and to have freedom to make their own choices.

In this chapter the life story of Eygló *Ebba* Hreinsdóttir is told in her own words (translated from Icelandic) to shed light on how normalisation influenced the lives and experiences of people with intellectual disabilities in Iceland during the latter half of the twentieth century. Ebba and I worked together as co-researchers for over 15 years. She was a wonderful person and friend and I deeply miss her. She made a significant contribution to co-researching and to the social history of intellectual disabilities in Iceland and internationally.

Ebba was born in 1950 and passed away in 2014. Her life story was published in Icelandic in 2010 (Hreinsdóttir with Stefánsdóttir, 2010). I have translated part of Ebba's story into English for this chapter. I also draw on the chapter we co-authored which was published in *Sexuality and Relationships in the Lives of People with Intellectual Disabilities* (Hreinsdóttir and Grétarsson with Stefánsdóttir, 2015).

Normalisation in the Nordic countries

The main contribution of the Nordic countries to the international development of policies and practices in services for people with intellectual disabilities has been normalisation. Bengt Nirje, a Swede, formulated a well-known exposition of the normalisation principle in 1969 (Nirje, 1969). However, the normalisation principle first appeared a decade earlier in Danish law. Niels Erik Bank-Mikkelsen, formerly director of the Danish Service for the Mentally Retarded, inserted the principle of the normalisation into the Danish Mental Retardation Act 1959 (Kirkebæk, 2001). At that time it was believed to be possible to normalise life in institutions and in the 1959 Act, the goal was that people with intellectual disabilities could have as close to normal conditions as possible at institutions, including going to school, work, and leisure activities inside the walls of the institution. In the beginning, normalisation was a programme for reforming and improving rather than replacing institutions. A decade later the normalisation concept became the grounds for criticisms of institutions for people with intellectual disabilities related to the disabling effects of long-stay institutions, poor living conditions and segregation (Tössebro et al, 2012).

Bengt Nirje's 1969 definition of normalisation emphasised rights to the same quality of life as non-disabled people and to participate fully in society. People with intellectual disabilities should have the same opportunities and conditions as non-disabled citizens, a normal life course and a normal rhythm of life. All of this should occur within normal environments and people with intellectual disabilities should not have to live in large institutions (Nirje, 1969; 1980).

Later, the German/American scholar Wolf Wolfensberger (1980) redefined normalisation, renaming it 'social role valorisation'. He argued that people with intellectual disabilities should be supported to take on valued social roles, which would enable them to live normal lives. Wolfensberger claimed that people with valued social roles are more likely to succeed in society but people who hold devalued positions in society are at risk of being treated badly, rejected by society, institutionalised and abused (Wolfensberger, 1980; 1998). Social role valorisation aims to work against the devaluation of people with intellectual disabilities by, for example, teaching them positive personal skills, training them to have highly valued work, and encouraging association with non-disabled individuals (Wolfensberger, 1980; 1998).

Both Wolfensberger's ideas and the Scandinavian principle of normalisation have been influential. Most disability research in the Nordic countries prior to the 1990s focused on issues associated with the Nordic welfare states with the aim to improve the quality of services (Gustavsson et al, 2005; Tössebro et al, 2012). However, the focus in Nordic disability research has been on services rather than on the experiences of people with intellectual disabilities. Their voices were missing. It could be argued that one of the reasons is that normalisation ideology was created and developed by non-disabled academics and professionals without the participation of people with intellectual disabilities (Walmsley, 2001).

Normalisation ideas, especially social role valorisation, have been criticised for focusing on changing people with intellectual disabilities instead of finding ways to eliminate disabling factors in society. Hollomotz (2011) pointed out that this approach does little to challenge oppression. Instead it puts pressure on individuals to learn adaptive behavior, as their acceptance into the community is conditional (p 39).

Furthermore, segregation remains common in the Nordic countries. A comprehensive review of recent developments in the Nordic countries, including Iceland, revealed that although all saw important reforms following the introduction of normalisation, large numbers still lived in segregated settings (Tössebro et al, 2012; Stefánsdóttir and Traustadóttir, 2015).

Normalisation and the story of Eygló *Ebba* Hreinsdóttir

This chapter explores how the ideology of normalisation influenced the life of Egló *Ebba* Hreinsdóttir, firstly how the institutional trap influenced her life after she moved out of an institution in 1976, how the staff at the group home sought to make Ebba a 'normal woman' and how she fought against it. Secondly the chapter aims to shed light on how the ideology of normalisation had a positive impact on the possibilities for people with intellectual disabilities to have relationships and get married even though aspects of the eugenic agenda were still alive, including the demand for childless marriage (Alþingi no. 18/1936; Wolfensberger, 1972).

The institutional trap and how to become a 'normal woman'

Eygló *Ebba* Hreinsdóttir was born on 19 December 1950. She lived with her family and siblings until she was 19, when she moved to an institution. Life at the institution was a terrible experience for Ebba:

> I lived with my family until my mother died and she couldn't die until she knew I was safe, and she thought that I was safe at the institution. She was a nice person and I love her deeply but she was like other people at this time. Everyone thought it was best for people like me to live in institutions. It was terrible to go to the institution. I remember being afraid all the time and I was ashamed and it is hard to live with the shame. I was so sad and angry those years and if I wasn't angry then I cried, so it was better to be angry. I am still angry but I have learned to live with it. At the institution I couldn't decide anything. The staff had their rules and everyone had to follow their rules. The worst of all was the label 'mentally retarded'. I didn't know that person who was labelled. It was not me.

Ebba lived at the institution for seven years until 1976 when she moved to the first group home established in Reykjavík.

> In 1976 I moved to the first group home in Iceland; we were six there in the beginning. I and my girlfriend Halla were the first to move, we were the pioneers. I don't like it when people are talking about all the pioneers and mean the staff and the people from the organisation. They forget us. If we didn't exist they wouldn't have been pioneers. It was much better to live at the group home than the institution. The staff treated us better. I got my own money but the staff did not understand us so well and we didn't get many opportunities there. I could never decide anything or have any control of my life. I was never asked and I hate it when I am not asked, I just get so angry. The staff still had lot of rules like at the institution and often they treated me like a child. In the weekend we had to be home by 12 o'clock in the evening, everyone had to have their meals at same time and so on. It was the same old story; if you have intellectual disabilities

people often treat you like you are in the third drawer. In the first drawer are these normal people. In the second drawer you have physically disabled people and in the third drawer you have people with intellectual disabilities. I did not want them to treat me like a child that needs care and supervision. The staff thought they were better than me. I want to make my own decisions but that was not possible at the group home.

John O'Brien (2005) claims that an institution is a trap for people with intellectual disabilities and getting out of the institution doesn't always mean getting out of the trap. As Ebba describes it, it was better to live in the group home, but the group home still had many institutional qualities built on inflexible rules and routines, where the staff bore all the responsibility for residents and made decisions for them. Ebba experienced belittling attitudes and restricted self-determination and was often viewed as an eternal child. Her testimony indicates that in the 1980s there was a gap between what actually happened and the normalisation principle (Nirje, 1969; 1980).

When Ebba and I were working on her life story we got permission to access medical records about Ebba when at the group home. As Atkinson (2004) observed, these types of records are often informative about the dominant views at a given point in history. We used fragments from Ebba's life-history as counter-narratives challenging the dominant discourse, reflecting among other things the influence of normalisation.

As stated earlier, normalisation ideas have been criticised as a construct created and developed by non-disabled academics and professionals without the participation of people with intellectual disabilities (Chappell, 1992; Walmsley, 2001). One of the consequences was that the practice of staff at the group home was dominated by normalisation ideas rather than Ebba's own views. It has also been argued that this led to the normalisation principle failing to recognise the nature of power relationships between professionals and people with intellectual disabilities rooted in the regime of the institutions where the staff had the power (Oliver, 1990).

Normalisation, especially social role valorisation (Wolfensberger, 1980), has also been criticised for seeking to change people with intellectual disabilities into so-called 'normal people', rather than calling into question their exclusion (Chappell, 1992). Part of that was they should accept their disability so that training could start at the right level (Wolfensberger, 1980). In Ebba's story the staff saw their role to train Ebba to become a 'normal woman'. Being herself was not good enough and she had to accept her disability. She describes that

Table 1: Ebba's story: contrasting narratives

Report written about Ebba by the staff and specialist at the group home, 1981	From Ebba's life story
The woman does not accept her disability and she is always reclaiming she is not 'mentally retarded'.	The staff at the group home were always telling me that I was 'retarded'. And the staff were always trying to control my life and always training me instead of helping me to be stronger.
She has to understand her limitation and face the fact that she is not like other people. She thinks she can do everything like people without disability. It is really important for her to accept her disability.	I have shown through my life I can do the same thing as people without disability can do. It just takes a longer time for me.
She does not listen to the staff and she protests constantly by breaking the house rules. It is possible to train Ebba to do a lot of things, like cooking and cleaning, but first she has to accept her disability and learn to control her behaviour.	Today I am living independently and I don't want any help from staff. If I had believed everything the staff said about me and to me I wouldn't be where I am today.

she doesn't like doing what was categorised as the typical women's role, for example cooking and sewing.

Ebba was a fighter and fought against these negative attitudes, and the staff who tried to boss her around, to achieve an independent life.

Sterilisation and a childless marriage

Many women were subject to involuntary sterilisation in the first half of the twentieth century (Tilley et al, 2012). Recent Icelandic research suggests that it was common practice to sterilise women with intellectual disabilities during the 1970s and 1980s, well after normalisation reached Iceland. It appears that sterilisation was usually carried out around time of transition: moving away from family to a group home, on the one hand, or from an institution to a group home on the other hand (Stefánsdóttir, 2014: Stefánsdóttir and Traustadóttir, 2015).

> In the beginning I wasn't going to talk about all the bad things that happened to me. The reason I didn't want to talk about the sterilisation and other bad things that have happened to me was because of shame. I was always ashamed and it is difficult to live with shame. I thought it was my fault because I was so stupid. After I started to tell my story and talk about the past, I realised it was not my fault and I should not be ashamed. It was not our fault we had to live in institutions or undergo sterilisation. It

was the government that decided how people with intellectual disabilities were treated. They should be ashamed. People should know that.

I was sterilised when I was fourteen. At that time, I lived with my parents and siblings. I didn't know about it until I was 26. At that time, I lived at the institution. The reason I learned about my sterilisation was because some of the other women at the institution were being prepared to undergo sterilisation. I asked: "Why not me?" And then the woman in charge of the institution had to tell me. I remember she told me that it was for our best interests to be sterilised. This was the year 1976 and at that time we were moving out from the institution into the first group home in Reykjavík. At that time my mother had passed away and it was difficult because I was so angry with her. I was not angry that I couldn't have children. I have never wanted to have a child, but I was angry because I didn't get the opportunity to decide for myself. I thought it was so humiliating to be sent to surgery, lied to and told your appendix had been removed. I didn't want to have children even after I got married.

After I started to talk about the institution and the sterilisation openly, I learned to accept these incidents and I have forgiven my mother and father. They were only doing what they thought was best for me at that time. They thought they were protecting me by sending me to an institution and sterilising me. I understand now that this was a historical phase, or I hope so. I also understand that this was not my fault; it was the government that decided to do such things to people. I don't think of it every day. I am over that now, but I think it is important to talk openly about sterilisation and how women with intellectual disabilities have been treated. It shouldn't be a secret.

As Ebba and many other women have described, sterilisation had a deep emotional impact (Stefánsdóttir, 2014). But what was most difficult for Ebba was that she was not trusted to make an autonomous decision concerning sterilisation. As stated in the normalisation principle, people with intellectual disabilities should have the opportunity to make their own decisions and have real choices (Nirje, 1980). But Ebba didn't have a choice when she was sterilised in the 1960s. Neither did her girlfriends ten years later as they had to undergo sterilisation as the price for moving out of the institution. The choice of remaining at the institution or being sterilised does not correspond to what is considered as a freely made choice.

Ebba was aware of the negative societal views about women with intellectual disabilities having children and the threat of losing custody. Even though the principle of normalisation advocated the need for significant shifts in attitude towards the sexuality of people with intellectual disabilities and emphasised the right to a sexual life and marriage, for many this excluded having children (Chapman et al, 2015). Wolfensberger (1972) considered social–sexual fulfilment as a right that must be achieved via childless marriage. The necessary sterility of such unions could be assured either by sterilisation or by contraception although the former should be voluntary. The argument often offered in defence of sterilisation was that it was for the best interest of the women, as Ebba pointed out in her story. This argument revolves around the idea that women are being protected (Brady, 2001). However, this is not the case. It can only protect them against one of the consequences, that is pregnancy (Hollomotz, 2011). From the perspective of the government, the sterilisation of women with intellectual disabilities protects society from the responsibility of taking care of and supporting parents with intellectual disabilities.

Ebba and her husband didn't have any option other than a childless marriage. Despite that, Ebba and Jonni had a happy marriage for over 20 years until she died in 2014.

> The best thing that happened in my life was that I met Jonni and we got married. That changed everything. I met Jonni in 1990. At that time I lived by myself in a small flat in a basement of the group home. I first met him on a winter's day when I slipped on the ice and fell into his arms. I have been there ever since. I am sure we were meant to meet each other on that day and be together forever. That was our destiny. Jonni and I fell in love and a few months later he moved into the flat with me and we got support from the staff at the group home. We got engaged on Jonni's birthday in 1990 in our flat. Jonni bought the rings and afterwards we went to Jonni's mother and told her. After that we went to his sister's place and waved our hands so she could see our rings, we were so happy and proud. She invited us for champagne and after that we went out for dinner, just the two of us. It was so romantic.
>
> After we first met I was anxious about telling Jonni about the sterilisation, but he thought it was all right. Jonni supports me and loves me like I am. It doesn't matter to him that I had to undergo sterilisation. Jonni and I have never had enough money to raise a child. Also I couldn't bear to have a child who would be taken away from me like many women with intellectual disabilities have experienced. We do not want to be dependent on assistance from staff or our families and we could not raise a child without support. I want to be independent, I always have. I think that Jonni would have liked more to have a child than I do, he loves children but he agrees that it would have been impossible for us to have children. We do everything together and although we do not always agree,

that's all right, we are best friends. Since we got married I can be myself and I know that he accepts me as I am and understands me. That makes all the difference.

Sexuality and relationships are an important part of human existence. Being loved and valued is of great importance as shown in Ebba's story. Ebba and Jonni emphasise the happiness that a good relationship can bring and that it can enable people to be more independent as a couple. Normalisation ideas had a significant impact on possibilities for people with intellectual disabilities to have relationships and get married. In that way, normalisation brought about positive change in Ebba's life.

Concluding comments

Even though normalisation and social role valorisation are criticised today, historically they brought significant improvements in the lives of people with intellectual disabilities. They played a huge role in deinstitutionalisation and, as Ebba described, it was a positive step towards her independence. However, her testimony shows that often there was a gap between her experiences and the normalisation principle which assumed that people with intellectual disabilities should have the right to self-determination and to a normal life (Nirje, 1969; 1980).

Despite improvements in community services in Iceland the majority of people with intellectual disabilities live in group homes or in assisted living with other people with intellectual disabilities. The domestic help people receive often has institutional qualities and there is a lack of access to mainstream society (Stefánsdóttir et al, 2018). The context in 2018 was better described as community presence rather than community inclusion.

Normalisation emphasised the right to a sexual life and marriage (Nirje, 1980). This brought a positive change in Ebba's life and in the lives of many other people with intellectual disabilities. But for Ebba it had to be a childless marriage. The status quo has been maintained and eugenics is still alive. Although involuntary sterilisation is no longer practised in Iceland, young women with intellectual disabilities are encouraged, by family members and carers, to undergo sterilisation as a form of contraception. It has also been argued that one of the consequences of the normalisation ideology is that the services and support system for people with intellectual disabilities in Iceland have normalised traditional gender roles (Björnsdóttir et al, 2017); being Ebba was not good enough, she had to become a 'normal woman'.

Iceland has ratified the CRPD and thereby recognises full human rights of people with disabilities. One of the key changes that the CRPD brings is that it treats disabled people as subjects capable of making decisions, not as objects to be managed or cared for. In 2018 Iceland was in the process of finalising draft legislation to bring Icelandic law into alignment with the Convention. Let's hope that in this process the Icelandic government and specialists learn from history and the experiences of people with intellectual disabilities. In Ebba's words: 'The government and the professionals should listen to us, we are the specialists in our lives'.

References

Alþingi no. 18/1936. *Lög um fávitahæli* [The Act on Sanctuaries].

Alþingi no. 47/1979. *Lög um aðstoð við þroskahefta* [The Act on Assistance to People with Intellectual Disabilities].

Alþingi no. 59/1992. *Lög um málefni fatlads fólks* [The Act on the Affairs of Disabled People].

Atkinson, D. (2004) 'Research and empowerment: involving people with learning difficulties in oral and life history research', *Disability and Society*, 19(7): 691–702, doi: 10.1080/096875904200084187

Atkinson, D. and Walmsley, J. (1999) 'Using autobiographical approaches with people with learning difficulties', *Disability & Society*, 21(2): 203–16.

Björnsdóttir, K., Stefánsdóttir, Á. and Stefánsdóttir, G.V. (2017) 'People with intellectual disabilities negotiate autonomy, gender and sexuality', *Sexuality & Disability*, 35(3): 295–311, doi: 10.1007/s11195-017-9492-x

Brady, S.M. (2001) 'Sterilization of girls and women with intellectual disabilities:past and present justifications', *Violence Against Women*, 7(4): 432–61, doi: 10.1177/10778010122182541

Chapman, R., Ledger, S. and Townson, L. with Docherty, D. (eds) (2015) *Sexuality and relationships in the lives of people with intellectual disabilities*, London and Philadelphia: Jessica Kingsley.

Chappell, A.L. (1992) 'Towards a sociological critique of the Normalisation principle', *Disability, Handicap & Society*, 7(1): 35–51, doi:10.1080/02674649266780041

Gustavsson A., Tøssebro, J. and Traustadóttir, R. (2005) 'Introduction: approaches and perspectives in Nordic disability research', in A. Gustavsson, R. Sandvin, R. Traustadóttir and J. Tøssebro (eds) *Resistance, reflection and change: Nordic disability research*, Lund: Studentliterature, pp 23–44.

Hollomotz, A. (2011) *Learning difficulties and sexual vulnerability: A social approach*, London and Philadelphia: Jessica Kingsley.

Hreinsdóttir, E.E. with Stefánsdóttir, G.V. (2010) *Ég var brautryðjandi. Lífssaga Eyglóar Ebbu Hreinsdóttir* [*I was a pioneer: The life history of Egló Ebba Hreinsdóttir*], Reykjavík: Guðrún V. Stefánsdóttir.

Hreinsdóttir, E.E. and Grétarsson, S.J. with Stefánsdóttir, G.V. (2015) 'Ebba and Jonni: This is our story', in R. Chapman, S. Ledger and L. Townson with D. Docherty (eds) *Sexuality and relationships in the lives of people with intellectual disabilities*, London: Jessica Kingsley, pp 65–77.

Karlsdóttir, U.B. (1998) *Mannkynbætur: Hugmyndir um bætta kynstofna hérlendis og erlendis 19. og 20. öld* [*Eugenics in the 19th and 20th century*], Reykjavík: Háskólaútgáfan.

Kevles, J. (1986) *In the name of eugenics*, London: Pelican.

Kirkebæk, B. (2001) *Normaliseringens periode*, København: SOCPOL Forlaget.

Nirje, B. (1969) 'The normalization principle and its human management implication', in R. Kugel and W. Wolfensberger (eds), *Changing patterns in residential service for the mentally retarded*, Washington, DC: President's Committee on Mental Retardation, pp 179–95.

Nirje, B. (1980) 'The normalization principle', in R.J. Flynn and K.E. Nitch (eds), *Normalization, social integration, and community service*, Baltimore, MD: University Park Press, pp 31–49.

O'Brien, J. (2005) 'Out of the institution trap', in K. Johnson and R. Traustadóttir (eds) *Deinstitutionalization and people with intellectual disabilities: In and out of institutions*, London: Jessica Kingsley, pp 259–73.

Oliver, M. (1990) *The politics of disablement*, Basingstoke: MacMillan.

Scheerenberger, R.C. (1983) *A history of mental retardation*, Baltimore, MD: Paul H. Brookes.

Stefánsdóttir, G.V. (2014) 'Sterilisation and women with intellectual disability in Iceland', *Journal of Intellectual and Developmental Disability*, 39(2): 188–97.

Stefánsdóttir, G.V. and Traustadóttir, R. (2015) 'Life histories as counter-narratives against dominant and negative stereotypes about people with intellectual disabilities', *Disability & Society*, 30(3): 368–80, doi: 10.1080/09687599.2015.1024827

Stefánsdóttir, G.V., Björnsdóttir, K. and Stefánsdóttir, Á. (2018) 'Autonomy and people with intellectual disabilities who require more intensive support', *Scandinavian Journal of Disability Research*, 20(1): 1–10, doi: https://doi.org/10.16993/sjdr.21

Tilley, E., Walmsley, J., Earle, S. and Atkinson, D. (2012) 'The silence is roaring: sterilization, reproductive rights and women with intellectual disabilities', *Disability & Society*, 27: 413–26, doi:10.1080/0968759 9.2012.654991

Tøssebro, J., Bonfils, I.S, Teittinen, A., Tideman, M., Traustadóttir, R. and Vesala, H. (2012) 'Normalization fifty years beyond: current trends in the Nordic countries', *Journal of Policy and Practice in Intellectual Disability*, 9(2): 134–46.

Walmsley, J. (2001) 'Normalisation, emancipatory research and inclusive research in learning disability', *Disability & Society*, 16(2): 187–205, doi: 10.1080/09687590120035807

Wolfensberger, W. (1972) *The origin and nature of our institutional models*, Syracuse: Center on Human Policy, Syracuse University.

Wolfensberger, W. (1980) 'A brief overview of the principle of normalization', in R.J. Flynn and K.E. Nitsch (eds) *Normalization, social integration and community service,* Baltimore, MD: University Park Press, pp 7–30.

Wolfensberger, W. (1998) 'A contribution to the history of Normalization with primary emphasis on the establishment of Normalization in North-America between 1967–1975', in R.J. Flynn and R.A. Lemay (eds), *A quarter-century of Normalization and social role valorization: Evaluation and impact*, Ottawa: University of Ottawa Press, pp 51–117.

NINE

Institutionalisation in twentieth-century New Zealand

Carol Hamilton

"We see life within a family as a fundamental right for
children as well as the best option. We see no place
for children in institutions solely on the grounds of
intellectual disability and believe that the appropriate
assistance in the home will help to sustain the
family. This will also be less costly to the State."
Craig et al, 1991, 22

"*E rere ki a puawai, e tipu ki a puwai, huia ka puwai.*"
["As the water flows and the new buds of
the forest arrive: So there is growth."]
Catherine Colebourne and the Waikato Mental Health
History Group, 2012, 146

Introduction

This chapter focuses on the impact of processes of institutionalisation
and deinstitutionalisation on the lives of people with learning/
intellectual disabilities in twentieth-century New Zealand.[1] Knowledge
about what happened during this period has been slow to emerge,
in part due to widespread acceptance within New Zealand society of
the idea of 'out of sight, out of mind' that surrounded the notion of
(intellectual) disability at this time. Later on, the desire for families
and communities to move on from institutional practices meant that
talk about what had happened was not encouraged. Further, many
who had been employed in institutions had signed Declarations of
Fidelity that promoted a code of silence about the nature of their
work. Gathering information about the experiences of the people
themselves has been difficult (Catherine Colebourne and the Waikato
Mental Health History Group, 2012, 227–9). However, the two
decades since 2000 have seen a growth in material about this still

sensitive area of New Zealand's social history. Records about individual patients have been archived and made available to the public. Personal stories are also accessible in a variety of on-line and text formats. As Craig et al (1991) suggest, the twentieth century saw a consolidation of the right of all intellectually disabled people to live within family and community groups and to access the support needed to do so. Yet to what degree the state actively supported deinstitutionalisation as a means of defraying costs rather than upholding rights is a question that remains open. I return to this at the end of the chapter.

Beginnings: institutionalisation in pre-twentieth-century New Zealand

European settlement in New Zealand began in earnest in 1840 and the first institution was built in Karori, Wellington in 1854. Between 1860 and 1900 large numbers of migrants, the majority from the United Kingdom (UK) and Ireland, arrived, many on assisted passages. Patterns of migration affected local Māori who struggled with the twin effects of European diseases (eg diptheria, tuberculosis, measles) and social and economic dislocation due to land confiscation (*Te Ara Encyclopaedia of New Zealand*, n.d. a). The rapid building of what were called asylums is testament to how quickly European ideas about physical and social 'fitness to belong' took root. Early asylums – Sunnyside (1863), Auckland (1867), Seaview (1872) and Nelson (1876) – followed a UK Victorian-style architecture: large, austere brick buildings in which 'the disturbed, the dangerous, the unpredictable' (Campion, 2012, 12), the ill and the socially vulnerable were confined. Yet asylum use took on a distinctly New Zealand dimension. Asylums offered a workable substitute for the loss, through migration, of wider family support networks. They also provided a one-stop-shop for both migrants and Māori that best utilised the skills of the few specialist medical practitioners (Brunton, 2003). Furthermore they provided employment for local community members (Kearns et al, 2012).

Asylums were initially overseen by provincial governments as no philanthropic or religious group was big enough to take on the financial responsibility. In 1876 responsibility was transferred to the newly formed Central Government in Wellington and subsequently held alongside the general hospital system under a Ministry of Health (MOH). State control provided the basis for management of confinement, care and rehabilitation in these settings for the next 80 years. Overcrowding soon became a problem. Two further asylums were built: Seacliffe Hall (1882), and Porirua (1887). Ashburn Hall, also built in 1882, was the first to be privately owned. It was located in Dunedin and operated alongside Seacliffe Hall, catering to the requirements of more well-to-do colonial families:

> [At Ashburn Hall] there is nothing in the cheery-looking block of buildings and picturesque surroundings to suggest the idea of a home for the insane.… Inside the buildings, as outside, there is really nothing, apart from the eccentricities of the occupants of the rooms, to indicate that Ashburn Hall is a home for the insane … (Torrance, 1890, 233)

Its opening indicated growing acceptance of institutionalisation as a means of managing the stigma involved in having a family member whose appearance and/or behaviour was deemed difficult or undesirable within the vision of New Zealand as a fit and moral society. Whether people with physical or cognitive disabilities were initially included within these euphemisms remains unclear. However, the issue of who was to be considered 'fit to belong' soon became such a pressing concern that in 1899 an Immigration Restriction Act prohibiting 'any idiot or insane person' (Office for Disability Issues, n.d.) from settling was put into place.

The twentieth century: the first 50 years

In the early years of the twentieth century a growing eugenics movement influenced key developments in the use of existing systems of institutionalisation in New Zealand. The science of eugenics, validated by the publication of *The Fertility of the Unfit* (Chapple, 1903), proposed that all human characteristics were heritable, with some more socially 'desirable' than others (Barker, 1983). The fertility of those with 'desirable' characteristics was to be encouraged, while the fertility of those with 'undesirable' characteristics was to be curbed. These ideas rapidly became moral imperatives, then government policies with real-time consequences for those who did not, or could not, 'fit in'. Segregation became the means of managing the behaviour of those who were considered to have the propensity to pass on undesirable traits, with 'protection, training and other benefits' available within 'a "well-regulated colony"' (Barker, 1983, 203), said to provide the most humane means of separating members of this group from their 'fitter' peers. Many with learning/intellectual disabilities became caught up in the practices of confinement that followed.

The New Zealand Plunket Society (NZPS), set up in 1907, attempted to regulate physical and social undesirability. Truby King, founder of the NZPS, was born in New Zealand, graduated from Edinburgh Medical School in 1886 and became medical superintendent of Seacliffe Hall in 1889 (Olsen, 1981). He believed that the high rate of infant mortality and the broader issue of social degeneracy could be reversed by training girls for motherhood:

> If women in general were rendered more fit for maternity, if instrumental deliveries were obviated as far as possible, if infants were nourished by their mothers, and boys and girls were given a rational education, the main supplies of population for our asylums, hospitals, benevolent institutions, gaols and slums would be cut off at the sources: further, a great improvement would take place in the physical, mental, and moral condition of the whole community ... (Olsen, 1981, 6)

The NZPS instituted a medicalised assessment of the development of infants and young children. Mobile Plunket-trained nurses were to go into homes to gather information about infant development. This information was then set alongside the normative infant/young child developmental standards of the time, against which decisions about 'fitness to remain' within the family were made. By 1914 branches of the NZPS could be found in the four main cities and in many smaller towns. By 1947 85% of non-Māori babies were within the Plunket system (Olsen, 1981). However, as Brookes (2014) points out, family members also played an important part when decisions to remove sometimes very young individuals to institutional care were made. These decisions were not always easy. Mothers in particular could be caught between their feelings for their child, the responses of other family members and prevailing cultural understandings of disability as 'a problem' to be solved by committing the child to an institution. Fathers were more likely to opt for institutionalisation (Brookes, 2014). The view that 'normal' children would be affected if the disabled child remained at home was widespread. Older children could be admitted when families were no longer unable to manage the individual at home. Factors leading to institutionalisation in these cases included 'changes in family circumstances, ill health or death of a parent or a change in behaviour of the family member' (Hoult, 2012, 54).

In 1911 the Mental Defectives Act provided political endorsement of the eugenics movement. Asylums became mental hospitals, and the classifying of specific degrees of 'deficiency from normal' was begun. Categorisation of defects underpinned the tightening-up of the nineteenth-century asylum system (Campion, 2012), while the indicators of deficiency – 'idiots, imbeciles, the feeble-minded and epileptics' (Campion, 2012, 16) – linked the categories to sets of personal characteristics or conditions. Idiots might have a physical disability as well as an IQ of between 20 and 50, an imbecile an IQ of between 50 and 70, possibly with no physical disability but would require care and control. The category of feeble-mindedness, or the group into which those who were 'incapable of competing on equal terms with their normal fellows' (Hoult, 2012, 54) were placed, was less clearly defined and used when individuals were deemed to require more control than care. These diagnostic models enabled medical practitioners to institutionalise 'defective' individuals. The 1911 Act also provided the groundwork for the subsequent Education Act 1914 – which obliged parents, teachers and police to report all categories of 'mentally defective' children to state authorities. During the 1920s two Committees of Inquiry, into Mental Defectives (1922) and Sexual Offenders (1925), raised concerns about the reproductive capacity of 'feeble-minded' children, bolstering the link between disability, delinquency and institutionalisation. A short-lived Eugenics Board was established in 1928. The Board was charged with keeping a register of those categorised under the Act as 'mentally defective persons' and to monitor resources used to manage them. It is not clear why the Board was disbanded, but some discomfort in the community about their tasks is indicated in this poem, 'A Mother's Lament', written by a local community member:

> "Oh Mother, save me from Dr Gray[2]
> 'Cause teacher says he's coming to-day
> And if I'm stupid he'll take me away."
> "I cannot save you, my little child,"
> His mummie said and her eyes were wild.
> "You belong to the State, you're no more my child!
> But Oh, my darling, don't stupid be
> Or he'll say we've tainted heredity,
> And must be eradicated – you and me!"
> (McClure, 2017)

By the mid-1930s, legislation, medical processes and social ideas about the confinement of those classified as unfit to live in a well-regulated society governed the operation of existing institutions. Four further institutions were built – Hokitika (1904), Tokanui (1912), Ngawhatu (1921) and Kingseat (1929). Cherry Farm opened in 1952. They comprised smaller villa–style ward accommodation within an overall complex. This change allowed for separation and management of psychiatric patients away from those considered mentally deficient (Dowland and Mackinley, 1985). Therapeutic programmes for psychiatric patients were set up and formal care and release plans put into place. These changes did not impact greatly on the treatment of the majority of those 'classified' as mentally deficient.

Tokanui Hospital, 1912–98

Tokanui was built in 1912, firstly to act as a central repository for chronic and incurable patients and to take the most challenging long-term and chronic cases from Porirua and Auckland. People with intellectual disability were more likely to become long-term residents, due to the lack of 'cure'. After a decade Tokanui began to admit patients directly. Individuals with intellectual disability were admitted into a specific ward of the hospital. They were housed in five ward areas. These received fewer resources and staffing than other wards and little therapy. Some wards were described as bare and featureless with toilet and bathing areas offering the bare minimum of privacy. Often care involved only the basic tasks of feeding, toileting and keeping residents clean. In some cases, training programmes were run for more severely disabled residents, usually due to the enthusiasm of a particular staff member who had an interest in working with intellectually disabled people. When this person moved on, the programmes ceased.

In 1959 people with intellectual disabilities accounted for around one fifth of the residents. When Tokanui closed in 1998 they were the majority.

Source: Colebourne and the Waikato Mental Health History Group, 2012.[3]

Admission of those with 'mental deficiency' to a hospital was made on the basis of a reception order given by a magistrate after an application was lodged. Applications were to be made by a person over 21 years of age. The grounds on which the applicant was deemed mentally defective were to be stated and the application itself accompanied by two medical certificates, issued not more than three days prior to the information being put before a magistrate (Campion, 2012).

Individuals admitted under the age of 21 required an application to be made to the Inspector-General of the MOH by a parent or guardian. A statutory declaration and two medical certificates were also needed. Individuals with intellectual disabilities could be admitted straight to a ward rather than through a reception area (Dowland and MacKinlay, 1985). The form of the induction depended on the informal protocols of the ward concerned.

> As part of the procedure all newcomers are given a bath or shower and put into night attire for a period of assessment … the reason for the night attire is to make them conspicuous until staff are familiar with them. Being put into pyjamas is a practice residents are not always happy with and one of the reasons new admissions are bathed is that it helps otherwise unwilling people to get into pyjamas … All property including clothes and valuables are taken away … Wards differ as to whether or not all newcomers are placed in pyjamas … The decision to come out of pyjamas often resting with the [ward] doctor (Dowland and MacKinlay, 1985, 14–15)

The management of 'mental deficiency' was the responsibility of the Mental Hospitals Department. Hospitals were inspected – in some cases inspection was required every three months – and an annual report produced. These documents included information about 'patient population … accommodation, farming operations, financial results, staff, medical superintendent's reports' (Campion, 2012, 17). Internal registers of admissions, boarders, discharges, escapees, restraints and seclusions, deaths and post-mortems, as well as weekly report books, case books and prescription books, were kept. Children and young people considered 'feeble-minded', or who had been made wards of the state, were more likely to be sent to a residential school as an alternative placement. These were established ostensibly to teach education and work skills to the young people involved. However, much depended on how the schools were run as to how much education was available. Early schools included Otekaieke (1908 – later called Campbell Park) for boys and Richmond (1916) for girls. Eventual release from the school was possible. Several psychopaedic units were also set up for more severely disabled children: Stoke Villas (1922), Templeton (1929) and, later on, Levin Training Farm and Colony (1945 – later called Kimberley Hospital). Release from psychopaedic units was far less likely.[4]

The twentieth century – the second 50 years

The second half of the twentieth century saw an increasing questioning of the efficacy of keeping disabled people in institutional settings. Knowledge of what had happened in Germany in the 1930s and 1940s when disabled and non-disabled people were subject to mass incarceration and execution, and New Zealand's commitment to the United Nations Universal Declaration of Human Rights in 1948 led to calls for the development of community care. In 1949 the Intellectually Handicapped Children's Parents Association (later IHC) was founded by Margaret and Hal Anyon, parents of a son with Down's Syndrome who wanted to see their disabled child educated, employed and living in the community. In the beginning IHC was concerned with securing community living for their members' young relatives with intellectual disability, who would live in hostel-style accommodation run by IHC-trained staff. This vision also provided a template for how community-based support could be provided for intellectually disabled adults who were resident in long-stay hospitals. However, as the process of deinstitutionalisation of physically and psychiatrically disabled people began, influential groups sought to retain the option of continued institutional placement for people with intellectual disabilities.

In 1952 a Government Consultative Committee was set up to consider the role of psychopaedic institutions. In 1953 the Aitken Report, named after the doctor who chaired the committee, was published (Stace, 2014). This recommended that intellectually disabled people continue to be housed in large 'mental deficiency colonies' and that the capacity of psychopaedic institutions, such as those at Levin (Kimberley) and Templeton, be increased. It further recommended that parents be encouraged to leave their disabled children in these institutions from about the age of five. Its influence was significant, as indicated in a report about residential capacity at Tokanui Hospital at the end of the 1960s.

> There is a constant demand for psychopaedic beds and a particularly heavy demand for the admission of children in the 5–15 age range … demand has remained high in recent years notwithstanding a very considerable build-up of subsidiary services such as occupation centres, hostels and sheltered workshops in local communities. (Department of Health, 1969, 100)

Case studies of admittance, 1950s–1970s

Robert – admitted to Kimberley in 1959, age 18 months. Left Campbell Park residential school in 1966, age 15:

> "I came [to Kimberley] when I was just a baby... I don't remember this time really well except that there was a lot of us and that even though I was small I know I had a mum and a dad and a sister. I cried for them but no-one came and eventually I stopped crying ... I know of stories of parents dropping their child off for the first time and then changing their minds on the way back home or after a week or two apart. Those parents couldn't just go back and pick up their baby. They had to battle the system and prove that they could look after their child before he or she could be released to them ..." (McRae, 2014, 14–23)

Alice – admitted to Kingseat Hospital in 1950, age 8. Left Carrington Hospital, age 48:

> "I saw Mum packing a suitcase in the dining room and I was just standing there watching. I said, what are you packing that suitcase for? Those look like my clothes, where am I going? And she said you're going to your Auntie Pats for a week's holiday. And the next morning Dad carried out the suitcase and put it on the back seat of the car ... when Dad had finished signing the papers they gave me a bath. I said I want to go home I don't like this place. They said, if you can behave yourself for a fortnight you can go home. And I was six months locked up in that observation ward." (Production SGDigital, 2015)

Norman – deemed low-grade feeble-minded. Admitted to Templeton, age 6. Went to work on a farm, age 18. Declared 'fit to live in normal society' in 1960, age 21:

> "It was a place where kids went to. Most had disabilities of some sort. They told me I would go to school there. I never got to go to school. Instead I worked on the farm. I had to look after the less abled, clean them up." (Smyth, n.d.)

Bev – as a ward of the state was admitted to Porirua Psychiatric Hospital in the 1960s, age 15. Left at an unknown date:

> "They'd put children locked up with these people in this ward ... we were attacked, we were treated absolutely terrible [She was subsequently given

electric shock treatment] ... I couldn't remember who I was and I couldn't remember why I was here ... when I woke up from it my throat was ... like I had something shoved down my throat." (Kearns et al, 2012)

Brent – admitted to Kimberley in 1972, age 2. Left when Kimberley closed in 1996.

"Mum and Dad say goodbye to me and they'll come back another day. I started to get a bit scared then. I didn't understand much, I was just a little boy then ... that's all I remember. 1972." (*Stuff*, 2014)

While demand for placements remained high, oversight of the living conditions of those with intellectual disabilities, never as rigorous as for those with other disabling conditions, became less and less thorough. Abuse and neglect, including 'physical, sexual, emotional, spiritual abuse, neglect and issues of control and restraint' (Mirfin-Veitch and Conder, 2017, 6) in the hospitals, units and residential schools were commonplace. Those who avoided abuse themselves had to witness the abuse and neglect of those they lived with. Some staff did what they could to keep residents safe in the hospitals and schools, and concerns about maltreatment were raised from the 1950s onwards. However, far too little was done to remedy the situation (DBI, 2008).

Robert
"... we were taken care of, fed and changed. But I don't remember being touched or cuddled like other kids are ... it was a lonely life. We grew up with hundreds of people around us but as a little boy I didn't know another human being. Not properly." (McRae, 2014, 15)

"Sometimes when you were in real trouble they'd take you to Villa 5 ... it was a nightmare and they would take you there as a warning that this was where you would end up if you didn't conform. I still remember being taken there and seeing this completely naked person who had an accident, being washed down with a fire-hose. He was screaming for them to stop... I was a small child back then." (McRae, 2014, 33–4)

Alice
"I used to get dragged down the corridor by staff by the feet and hair and they throw me into a seclusion room there ... and I screamed and screamed and screamed at them, pleaded with them to let me out ... the nurses used to look into you to see what you were up to. If they saw you were

up to no good they'd get reinforcements and unlock the door and come in with a couple of hypodermic needles." (Production SGDigital, 2015)

Norman

"I was abused at Templeton. I was beaten by staff and patients. Life there was hell ... sexually abused, ahh, sodomised, you know. I suppose you could say that it continued on – not just only me but I think a lot of other people too....You don't forget, doesn't matter how much counselling you have ..." (Smyth, n.d.)

Robert

"Don't get me wrong. There was some good staff .... they gave me books and toy animals from cereal packets and sometimes they took me home to their places at the weekend. I used to cling to those staff but always, in the end, they'd walk out of my life ..." (McRae, 2014, 32)

Alice

"I had a lot of nurse friends that stuck up for me ..." (Production SGDigital, 2015)

While debates for and against institutional care continued, wider societal views about the capacity of young people with intellectual disabilities to learn were changing. Media, including locally produced films, were instrumental in raising public awareness about the capacity of children with intellectual disabilities to learn if given the chance. Commentary from a 1960s film documentary about training offered to intellectually disabled young people in three psychopaedic institutions – Templeton, Ngawhatu and Kimberley – indicates how community views about ability and members of this group were beginning to alter. This documentary included the follow statement alongside footage of intellectually disabled children learning in a new on-site training centre:

> [these institutions] ... are caring for 1,500 patients, most of them children ... yet the patients are not necessarily physically ill. The children here are sick, yes, but the sickness is locked away inside their heads ... these are inspiring places, where the close mysterious horizons of the mentally retarded's world are slowly clearing. (New Zealand National Film Unit, 1964)

Further questions about the efficacy of institutional placement for intellectually disabled people saw the movement to reintegrate individuals from institutions gain more momentum from the early 1970s (Hoult, 2012). Having developed a strong information and advocacy role for families and at government level, IHC applied for government funding to purchase and manage family homes in suburban towns. By the late 1970s it had become a powerful, nation-wide organisational network that was almost sole provider of residential services for people with intellectual disabilities. IHC was an enthusiastic adopter of the principles of normalisation, 'letting the retarded obtain an existence as close to normal as possible' (Nirje, 1969, 3). This idea became a cornerstone belief for IHC service delivery (Craig et al, 1991). Yet by the end of the 1980s, deinstitutionalisation processes across the country remained slow. The lack of a national plan for the reduction of numbers living in institutions coupled with the lack of community-based placements for those leaving presented particular barriers, as this excerpt from an IHC report shows.

> The 550 houses at present owned by the Society will be insufficient if there is a substantial number of transfers of residents from psychopaedic institutions to IHC services. (Craig et al, 1991)

Other limiting factors included transition costs and the fiscal implications of supporting a diminishing number of people left in the institutions (Craig et al, 1991). At the time, a long-stay supplement of $88.44 (NZ$158.00 in 2017) per day was paid to local area health boards who held contracts to support individuals in long-stay accommodation. Shifting individuals out of institutional care represented a considerable loss to these providers. Supporting people to leave was further complicated by a government proposal to shift responsibility for all funding and coordination of services from the MOH to the Ministry of Social Welfare. This proposal took a number of years to action (PSA, 1990, 3). Further, the strong belief of some parents/guardians of the benefits of institutional care made it difficult for some residents to leave (Craig et al, 1991). Finally, some institutions were significant local employers, leading to local pressure to keep them. Waiting left some staff in limbo; one staff member reported remembering a discussion about the closure of Kimberley at her interview 17 years earlier (DBI, 2008). Institutional staff were seen as not having the right philosophy and skills to work in community services, and advertised community-based positions were not open to them (DBI, 2008). As a response, the MOH set up guidelines for ensuring how full community support for deinstitutionalised intellectually disabled people was to be actioned. These included that people be accommodated in 'homes … that look like others in the neighbourhood, and for locations [to be] close to a wider range of community resources' (Harnett et al, 1988, 3).

Some areas made more resettlement progress than others. In the Waikato region 40 residents of Tokanui Hospital had left by the end of the 1980s, while in Otago 'only 12 of the 140 people identified at Cherry Farm as having an intellectual disability have been transferred' (Craig et al, 1991, 3). For those able to leave, life was, in some ways, very different. Yet some indicators suggest that the people themselves had little option about who they lived with and how they chose to live their lives.

Tokanui Hospital Group, Community Home Evaluation, 1988

A Community Home Evaluation team visited two community-based residence initiative pilot projects in the Waikato region. After an extensive review of the physical environment, support structures and the programmes available to the people from Tokanui living in the residences, the evaluation team concluded that the transition process from the institution had been largely successful.

5.1 Routines

In general the daily routines of the homes followed patterns typical of most New Zealanders. Bed times, waking up, mealtimes, showers and household chores were completed at times in keeping with average New Zealand families. Rigid hospital routines have not been transferred to the community setting as evidenced one Friday night when the evaluators went shopping and banking with the ____ Road residents and sat down to a greatly appreciated meal of fish and chips at around 8.15pm.

5.6 Personal Wellbeing of Clients

Individual health needs were closely attended to at both community homes, medication reviews were carried out regularly by appropriately qualified people. The standard of dress of the residents was particularly pleasing. This is important if the residents' presentation in the community is to enhance their dignity as adults. The staff of both houses are to be congratulated for the high standards they have achieved in this area.

Source: Harnett et al, 1988, 8–10.

There is no question that community involvement had improved the lives of people released from long-stay hospital care, yet questions remained. Hospital routines were not transferred but, in their place, dominant ideas about how the average New Zealander spent their day came to govern significant aspects of their lives. These could be equally restricting. This statement was made at an early conference about the rights and needs of disabled people:

> "... their rights to normal living are offered on the one hand and taken away with the other e.g. one of the conditions of semi-independent flatting, which is a good step in the right direction, for women at one branch, is that they must either have a tubal ligation or a hysterectomy. In another case a woman who was forced to undergo these measures now wants to marry and have children. No one is prepared to tell her she can't have children, but she is encouraged to get married and try anyway." ('The Handicapped: Rights, Needs, Services' seminar, 1979, 35)

Health and well-being were more closely attended to than they had been previously, but how much emotional support for trauma experienced while living in institutional care was needed or offered remains an open question:

> She conveyed how she re-lived the trauma of her feelings and experiences while in State care through her dreams: "Sometimes I dream about the hospitals I have been in. It can happen any time. When I dream about those places the dreams always wake me up. They are bad dreams. I wake up scared that I am still there." (Hunter, 1997, 12)

By the last decade of the twentieth century over 11,000 people were receiving community-based residential support (PSA, 1990). Community groups began grappling with how to manage the support requirements of two distinct cohorts – younger people who had never experienced institutional care, and older people who had been through this system. IHC had been at the forefront of the deinstitutionalisation movement, but was increasingly seen as an organisation that could not support both groups effectively.

By the end of the twentieth century how intellectually disabled people were to be supported to live in their local community had become an issue of national priority. In 2000, a National Advisory

Committee on Health and Disability was set up under sections 11 and 13 of the New Zealand Public Health and Disability Act 2000 to provide independent advice to the Minister of Health on a range of issues. The committee led a nationwide consultation process prior to publication in 2003 of the first comprehensive vision for community-based support for intellectually disabled people, the *To Have An 'Ordinary' Life – Kia Whai Oranga 'Noa'* policy document (Ministry of Health, 2003). The process included 10 facilitated focus groups of up to 10 intellectually disabled people who spent two days discussing issues that were important to them (Ministry of Health, 2003). Family/Whanau and service sector focus groups were also held. *To Have An Ordinary Life* recognised that 'all people, whatever their level of impairment, have the same fundamental human needs and expectations' (Ministry of Health, 2003, 2) as their non-disabled peers. Its 23 recommendations outlined changes needed including: needs assessment, service coordination, survice purchasing, and service delivery. To deliver on people's aspirations about where, how and with whom they live, publication was followed by closure of the last psychopaedic institution, Kimberley Hospital, in 2006.

Conclusion

The success of the deinstitutionalisation movement in New Zealand was largely due to the persistent advocacy of groups of family members and support personnel who wanted to see a move away from regimes of custodial care, and the establishment of high-quality and respectful community-based service systems. There was much to be optimistic about the goal of full community membership in the early years of the twenty-first century. *To Have An Ordinary Life* (Ministry of Health, 2003) captured the aspirations of parent and advocacy groups. It also provided a vision for people to tell their stories and to record what they want in their lives. However, the late twentieth-century difficulties associated with management and funding of the support needed to achieve these goals persisted into the twenty-first century. As Joseph and Kearns (1997) remarked soon after the closure of Tokanui Hospital, 'institutions have been easily closed, but less easily replaced' (p 187). This statement is reflected in the contemporary educational, social and health problems that remain embedded in the support systems on which intellectually disabled people and their family members must rely. These include ongoing difficulties with assessment and funding of individual educational and social needs, the difficulties some people have in exercising choice and control over aspects of their lives, and the lack of real choice among a number of service providers for those leaving home as young adults. Competition for social welfare funding is fierce and community-based services are particularly vulnerable in periods of fiscal austerity. New support service initiatives such as the Enabling Good Lives Demonstration[5] are a welcome move to improve both support and funding options. However, funding for projects connected to this Demonstration are allocated on year-by-year cycles, thus long-term funding is not guaranteed. What happens when funding is withdrawn and why the full inclusion of intellectually disabled people is so hard to achieve are questions that have no ready answers. What is important is that we do not forget what happened in the past and that the lessons that can be taken from what went on then can be used to inform what needs to happen in the future.

Postscript: Email from Dr Carol Hamilton to The Royal Commission of Inquiry into Historical Abuse in State Care, 26 April 2018

Carol:
> ... do the terms of enquiry include State Care in residential facilities? Reason for asking is that I'm writing a book chapter about institutionalisation processes – it's an international publication – and would like to include that this enquiry is taking into consideration past practices of ID [intellectually disabled] people's care in institutional settings.

Gordon [for the Royal Commission]:
... the Royal Commission of Inquiry into Historical Abuse in State Care will include consideration of care provided to people with Intellectual Disabilities in residential facilities such as Kimberley and Tokanui. I hope this clarifies the matter for you.

Appendix

Approximate number of people in New Zealand with an intellectual disability in 1991

South Island

Braemar/Ngawhatu	208
Cherry Farm	169
Gore Hospital	9
Seaview	69
Templeton	550

North Island

Kimberley	492
Lake Alice	3
Mangere	342
New Plymouth	24
Porirua	139
Tokanui	350

Total 2,439

With families or in their own homes	5,300
In IHC homes	3,000
In Hohepa Homes	150
Mr Tabor Trust Homes	41
Other	309

Total current estimate 11,000 (approx.)

Psychiatric hospitals

Carrington, Kingseat, Raventhorpe, Tokanui, Lake Alice, Porirua, Ngawhatu, Seaview, Sunnyside, Cherry Farm

Source: Craig et al (1991), 32.

Notes

[1] The Treaty of Waitangi was signed in 1840 when NZ became a British colony.

[2] Dr Gray, originally from Scotland, proposed severe eugenics-inspired measures for the registration and isolation of 'mental defectives' in New Zealand. He became head of New Zealand's mental hospitals in 1927.

[3] The Waikato Mental Health History Group was set up by Associate Professor Catharine Colebourne from the University of Waikato as part of an oral history project into mental health in the Waikato region of New Zealand. Tokanui Hospital was the fourth-biggest long-stay psychiatric and intellectual disability institution in the country and was situated outside of Te Awamutu. Many local people were connected over time with the hospital, which was one of the biggest employers in the region.

[4] New Zealand was unique in offering a three-year qualification in psychopaedic nursing. This was an allied mental health qualification for people wishing to work with people with intellectual disabilities. The qualification was completed 'on the job' and was disestablished in 1989.

[5] Information about the Enabling Good Lives Project can be found at www. enablinggoodlives.co.nz

References

Barker, D. (1983) 'How to curb the fertility of the unfit: the feeble-minded in Edwardian Britain', *Oxford Review of Education*, 9(3), 197–211.

Brookes, B. (2014) *Family emotional economies and disability at birth.* Retrieved from: https://remedianetwork.net/2014/08/08/family-emotional-economies-and-disability-at-birth/#comments

Brunton, W. (2003) 'The origins of deinstitutionalisation in New Zealand', *Health and History*, 5(2), 75–103.

Campion, M. (2012) 'Mental health and legal landscapes', in C. Colebourne and the Waikato Mental Health History Group (eds) *Changing times, changing places: From Tokanui Hospital to Mental Health Services 1910–2012,* Hamilton, New Zealand: Half Court Press, pp 27–53.

Chapple, W.A. (1903) *The fertility of the unfit*, New Zealand: Whitcombe and Tombs.

Colebourne, C. and the Waikato Mental Health History Group (eds) (2012) *Changing times, changing places: From Tokanui Hospital to Mental Health Services 1910–2012*, Hamilton, New Zealand: Half Court Press.

Craig, M., Jones, S., Lovelock, G. and Young, V. (1991) *Report of the IHC Review Working Party – prepared for The Hon Jenny Shipley, Minister of Welfare,* February 28. Retrieved from https://waikato-primo.hosted.exlibrisgroup.com/primo-explore/fulldisplay?docid= 64WAIKATO_ALMA2154578400003401&context=L&vid =64WAIKATO&lang=en_US&search_scope=WAIKATO_ ALL&adaptor=Local%20Search%20Engine&tab=waikato_ all&query=any,contains,Report%20of%20the%20IHC%20 review%20working%20party&sortby=rank&facet=rtype,exclude, newspaper_articles&facet=rtype,exclude,reviews

DBI (Donald Beasley Institute) (2008) *The Kimberley Report.* Retrieved from: www.donaldbeasley.org.nz/assets/Uploads/publications/DBI-KimberleyReports-Staff.pdf

Department of Health (1969) *A review of hospitals and related services in New Zealand.* Retrieved from: www.moh.govt.nz/notebook/ nbbooks.nsf/0/5C05938CA2D6B6EA4C2565D70018F567/$fi le/36151.pdf

Dowland, J. and McKinlay, R. (1985) *Caring, curing and controlling: An outsider's look at life and work in New Zealand Psychiatric Hospitals.* Retrieved from: http://www.moh.govt.nz/notebook/nbbooks.nsf/ 0/1fe89b7787104fab4c2565d70018931a/$FILE/Caring,%20curing. pdf

Harnett, F., Robertson N. and Smith, C. (1988) 'An evaluation of the establishment of group community homes for people with intellectual handicaps, Tokanui Hospital'. Access at University of Waikato Library, New Zealand Collection.

Hoult, A. (2012) 'Intellectual disability: the patient population in Tokanui', in C. Colebourne and the Waikato Mental Health History Group (eds) *Changing times, changing places: From Tokanui Hospital to Mental Health Services 1910–2012,* Hamilton, New Zealand: Half Court Press, pp 53–67.

Hunter, A. (1997) *My life,* Dunedin, NZ: Donald Beasley Institute.

Joseph, A.E. and Kearns, R.A. (1996) 'Deinstitutionalization meets restructuring: the closure of a psychiatric hospital in New Zealand', *Health & Place,* 2(3), 179–89.

Kearns, R., Joseph, A.E. and Moon, G. (2012) 'Traces of the New Zealand psychiatric hospital: unpacking the place of stigma', *New Zealand Geographer,* 68(3), 175–86.

McClure, T. (2017) 'The dark, unknown story of eugenics in New Zealand', 6 December. Retrieved from: https://www.vice.com/ en_nz/article/7xw9gb/the-dark-unknown-story-of-eugenics-in-new-zealand

McRae, J. (2014) *Becoming a person*, Nelson: Craig Potton Publishing.

Ministry of Health (2003) *To Have An 'Ordinary' Life – Kia Whai Oranga 'Noa'*. Retrieved from: www.moh.govt.nz/notebook/nbbooks.nsf /0/767269395A2349ABCC256DA2007133FD/$file/To-have-an-ordinary-life.pdf

Mirfin-Veitch, B. and Conder, J. (2017) *'The institutions are places of abuse': The experiences of disabled children and adults in state care*. Retrieved from: www.hrc.co.nz/files/3415/0103/3949/Institutions_ are_places_of_abuse-__The_experiences_of_disabled_children_and_ adults_in_State_care_.pdf

New Zealand National Film Unit (1964) *One in a thousand*. Retrieved from https://www.nzonscreen.com/title/one-in-a-thousand-1964.

Nirje, B. (1969) 'Changing patterns in residential services for the mentally retarded'. Retrieved from: www.disabilitymuseum.org/ dhm/lib/detail.html?id=1941&page=all

Office for Disability Issues (n.d.) *History of disability in New Zealand*. Retrieved from: https://www.odi.govt.nz/about-disability/history-of-disability-in-new-zealand/

Olsen, E. (1981) 'Truby King and the Plunket Society: an analysis of a prescriptive ideology', *New Zealand Journal of History*, 15(1), 3–23.

Production SGDigital (2015) *Alice, 50 Years Under the System*, 23 April. Retrieved from: www.youtube.com/watch?v=l4yM_-KxKIY

PSA (Public Service Association) (1990) 'Government turns services to the intellectually handicapped upside down', June. Copies available on request from PSA National Office, PO Box 3817, Wellington, New Zealand.

Smyth, G. (n.d.) *Out of sight, out of mind*. Retrieved from: https:// gerardsmyth.nz/works/out-sight-out-mind/

Stace, H. (2014) *Cool Asylum: Porirua Hospital Museum*. Retrieved from: https://publicaddress.net/access/cool-asylum-porirua-hospital-museum/

Stuff (2014) 'Stepping into the past – The Kimberley Centre', 27 December. Retrieved from: www.stuff.co.nz/national/64490246/ stepping-into-the-past-the-kimberley-centre

Te Ara Encyclopaedia of New Zealand (n.d. a) 'Story: History of immigration'. Retrieved from: https://www.teara.govt.nz/en/ history-of-immigration/page-10

Te Ara Encyclopaedia of New Zealand (n.d. b) 'Story: Contraception and sterilisation'. Retrieved from: https://www.teara.govt.nz/en/ contraception-and-sterilisation/page-4

'The Handicapped: Rights, Needs, Services' seminar (1979), held 19 and 20 November at Massey University, Palmerston North, New Zealand.

Torrance, J.A. (1890) *Picturesque Dunedin: Or Dunedin and its neighbours.* Dunedin: Mills, Dick and Co. Retrieved from: http://nzetc.victoria.ac.nz/tm/scholarly/tei-BatPict-t1-body1-d9-d6.html

TEN

'My life in the institution' and 'My life in the community': policies and practice in Taiwan

Yueh-Ching Chou

Introduction

This chapter considers the history of people with intellectual disabilities in Taiwan in the twentieth century. It opens with an account of the historical and political context, before considering the life stories of three Taiwanese citizens with intellectual disability.

Historical and political context in Taiwan

After the Second World War, Japan left Taiwan, which it had colonised for 50 years. Subsequently Taiwan was governed under martial law by the Republic of China (ROC). Following the Chinese Civil War, the People's Republic of China (PRC) took power in China and the ROC government moved to Taiwan in 1949. Taiwan has been called 'the state of the Miracle' (Dessus et al, 1995; Gold, 1986) because of its economic development in the 1970s and 1980s. However, social welfare, including disability welfare, was not part of the government's bureaucracy until 1980 when three welfare laws – the law for the elderly, the social assistance law and the law for the disabled – were enacted and implemented.

The year martial law was abolished, 1987, was a landmark for all Taiwanese people including disabled people. Non-profit organisations working for vulnerable people were legalised; welfare for disabled people was promoted by various non-governmental organisations (NGOs), following public campaigning and lobbying that sought to mobilise assistance for disabled people. In the 1990s, as a result of these efforts, the welfare law for the disabled was amended (eg in 1990 and 1997), and additional resources were allocated in particular for the establishment of institutions for people with intellectual disabilities.

NGOs were integrated as major partners with the official welfare system (Hsiao and Sun, 2000; Chou et al, 2006). Privatisation became the major trend in welfare services in the 1990s; most institutions were established and managed by NGOs during that period.

Taiwan became a democratic country with a president elected by the people in 1997, and 2000 saw the first transformation of government from the old party, established in China, to a new party, established in 1986 in Taiwan. As a result of democratisation, the government was obliged to concern itself with social needs. Meanwhile, Taiwan was influenced by the welfare experiences of Western and other East Asian countries like Japan. These influences led, for example, to the creation of the independent living movement for people with intellectual disabilities in Taiwan in 2001.

Since the passage of the Disability Act in 1980, welfare support for people with disabilities in Taiwan includes both services and financial entitlements, based on the degree of disability (mild, moderate, severe or profound) and family income. Recipients of disability benefits must go through official registration based on their medical diagnosis or, since 2012, the International Classification of Functioning, Disability and Health (ICF) (Chou and Kröger, 2017). The individual is given a certificate, an intellectual disabilities card, that shows her/his eligibility for disability benefits and services. Local authorities in Taiwan may provide a monthly family subsidy and a range of services including a subsidy for using residential services.

Institutionalisation

Taiwan has a population of 23 million people, and 100,000 persons have been identified as having an intellectual disability (4.3 per thousand). In Taiwan, care for family members is a family responsibility and required by the Civil Code. Most (90%) people with intellectual disabilities live with their families. Nevertheless, the number of people living in institutions is growing (Chou and Schalock, 2007; Chou, 2017).

The earliest registered institution providing residential care services for orphans and children labelled as mentally retarded was founded in 1952 (Department of Social Affairs, MOI, 2002). Before 1952, efforts to aid persons with an intellectual disability were carried out by religious groups and private individuals. Until the 1990s charities were not registered by the government. Before then, facilities providing services were all large, the minimum unit size being 30. This was changed to 20 in 1990. The first 'community home' (for

20 to 30 people) was organised in 1990 in Taipei City by parents. Since 1997, when the Disability Act was amended, group homes have been established for fewer than 30 people. Ordinary homes in the community for six or fewer residents were launched in 2004, sponsored by central government (Chou et al, 2008).

Deinstitutionalisation has never been state policy in Taiwan. Many parents still prefer institutions, and the voices of people with intellectual disabilities are still unheard. Although Taiwan is not a member of the United Nations, the UNCRPD (United Nations Convention on the Rights of Persons with Disabilities) Implementation Act was passed in 2014. This means that the Taiwan government has to undertake the general obligations as stated in Article 4 of the UNCRPD. The government invited international disabled activists to Taiwan in autumn 2017 as international reviewers for the State Report of CRPD. Article 19 of the CRPD became an important mechanism for the movement supporting people's right to choose where they live.

Life stories

Chang's story: a whole life protected

I knew Chang when I worked at FUGEI Institution in 1983. I interviewed him at a room in SUN Institution, where he lived until 1991.

Chang

Chang[1] was born in 1968. He was 49 when I interviewed him. He was abandoned when he was born, and police sent him to a homeless shelter. In 1977, aged nine, he went to live in FUGEI,[2] an institution for children and youth with intellectual disabilities. Chang moved to SUN[3] when he was 23. He was sterilised[4] when he lived in FUGEI, a requirement for people living in the institution before the 2000s. SUN also had this regulation until 2002. In 1991 Chang, along with 11 other men, moved to a 'Community Home'[5] owned by SUN.

> "I do not know which year I was born. Teachers[6] know how old I am. I do not have father and mother; I am an orphan. I have Teacher Yen, she is our teacher. During New Year, I went to K City, Teacher Yen drove me there. I miss Teacher Yen and the teachers of FUGEI. Teacher Yen is busy; she did not come to see me. I want to talk with Teacher Yen and see whether she can take me home. Teacher Yen came to see me and said

that I am 'quai-quai' [meaning good and obedient]. Many teachers are there and I want to see them. I live in SUN for a long time but I do not know how many years.

I am up at six o'clock and I clean teeth, wash face, shave and eat breakfast. I live in Community Home. I like to live in Community Home more than here [SUN Institution]. Community Home for me is good to sleep, because there we have spring bed and the room is bigger. Here many persons live together. Community Home is 'outside', air is better; we have shops to buy things. In the institution you cannot go out; it is locked. Community Home is good, taking a walk or go to temple for worship is allowed. We just tell teacher I am going out to buy things. Then he knows.

We eat lunch here and take a nap here. We come to here for breakfast. In the evening we go back to Community Home for dinner. I sleep in a room with Song. We have many rooms. Y-Chia and Y-Hau went back to their home. At Community Home we have TV. I use my money to buy TV in my room. Here there is no TV. We [Chang and the residents of the Community Home] stay at Community Home during weekend, we watch TV there, and clean toilet. So we do not come back here during the weekend. During the New Year, we move here, sleeping for 10 days. They [other residents having family] go home, but we do not. After the New Year, we move back to Community Home.

I clean the first floor. I clean the toilet at the second floor. Toilets all are cleaned by me. I also help to clean the farm. Teacher K is kind to me. He is my teacher; Y-Ling is also his case and he has six 'cases'.

Today I should go to MM Shoes Factory for work. But I do not need to go now. I work at the MM, making shoes. I work one day a week, no work.[7] Boss says no work due to business recession. I bike to the factory by myself. I finish my work at five o'clock. The teacher saves my salary in the post office. If I want to have 200 dollars to buy things, I go to teacher to have money.

Y-Chia is my good friend; he is not here now. Y-Chia lives in Taipei. Y-Chia and Y-Hau go to Thailand for fun; their sister takes them home. Y-Chia and Y-Hau go home for fun. I do not know when they will be back.

Tomorrow we are going to take High Speed Railway (HSR). I do not know where we are going. We have five persons go together. I am very happy to take HSR. I like to take HSR, to go to shopping mall, to go to Carrefour to buy things. I buy fast noodle, cookies, and drinks. Every Friday teacher takes us to buy things at the Carrefour. I have never been there by myself. We need to take car to Carrefour. There we can eat fried noodle, rice; we can eat many things.

I am not married. I want to marry. Y-Mei is my friend and classmate. Y-Mei lives here in the women's building; she does not live with me. She wants me to send her a ring, she says I can marry her during the New Year. Her mother takes her home, and then takes her back. I have money to marry her. If she gives birth to a baby who will call me father. We do not kiss, I hold her hands to go out for fun and for eating. I did not yet go to teacher to have money for buying ring. I have gone to see the ring. I am happy to marry with Y-Mei; our teachers all know."

Notes:

[1] All names have been changed.

[2] FUGEI was established by a private charity in 1970 for children aged between eight and 16. It was transferred to become a public institution for children in 1978. Now it is an institution for adults, and is directed by central government.

[3] SUN was designated an 'Education and Nursing Institution', the term used for intellectual disability institutions in Taiwan since the 1970s. SUN became one of three institutions run by central government for adults with intellectual disabilities in 1999. SUN is a residential campus, distributed into 10 units, in a rural area. Currently 450 residents, 350 men and 100 women, live there. Between 40 and 50 people share accommodation based on their level of disability.

[4] The Taiwan Genetic Health Law 1984 states that anyone diagnosed with a genetic disease or mental illness may choose to be sterilised (Chou and Lu, 2011).

[5] SUN bought this house, with two units. Six men share a unit, which has three bedrooms, each bedroom shared between two. Twelve men share the living room and kitchen. The house is only for men who have paid work outside the institution.

[6] In Taiwan, service users and family call the staff working with them 'Teacher'. It implies that the staff are role models who should be respected by service users and family.

[7] When Chang moved to SUN, aged 23, he started working at this shoe factory. Now most of the factory has moved to China.

Jenny's story: just doing what she is told

Jenny

Jenny was born in 1960 and has lived in SUN Institution since 1993 after her husband died in 1990. She shares the accommodation with 49 women (aged 21–76) and shares a bedroom with three roommates. She attended school until fifth grade. Her mother had a hearing impairment and she was cared for by her grandmother until her death. Both Jenny's father and husband were veterans.[1] Her two children were born in 1984 and 1987 and were adopted.

"I forgot how old I am; I need to ask my teacher. My two kids were given to others. They are girls; it has been long time ago. I do not know where they live. I do not know how old they are. I forgot all these things. My brother has told me that I should not think about them, he wants me to forget them.

My brother is busy and he has no time to visit me. My brother takes me home and takes me out for fun and for eating, for buying things; he buys me something. I phone my brother; he needs to work and he has no time to receive my phone. I cannot remember my brother's telephone number; teachers know. My brother came to visit me on Saturday; I am very happy my brother come to see me. During New Year, my brother takes me home; I am very happy. He drives me out for fun. He worries I am hungry and he buys me food. He wants me to sleep, I sleep. He says to me for taking a shower, I take a shower. The thing I like most is that my brother takes me home, comes to visit me, telephones me, and takes me to worship father and mother.[2]

My husband died long time ago. He was older than me. He was from a foreign province.[3] He was an old taro and my father was an old taro too. My father died. My mother died because of illness. I have a sister; she never comes to see me.

Grandmother died; she took care of me. I miss her. When I was a kid she took good care of me and she raised me up. Grandmother cooked for me; I do not know how to cook. When grandmother sent me here [SUN]; I was crying. Grandmother said that my husband died and I had no person to take care of me.

I had been sterilised. Grandmother said that I am not able to raise a kid. I gave birth to two kids and I was sterilised. Grandmother did it.

I have been here [in the institution] for a long time. I forgot how old I was when I came here. I am happy here; two teachers take good care of me very well. I live in T unit and my good friends live in S unit. I help teachers to wash dishes, dry clothes, help classmates changing diapers. I go to take bakery class and join drum social group. Teachers take us out for fun; I am happy. Teacher wakes me up in the morning. Teacher tells me to eat breakfast. For dinner I eat rice; food is good. I watch TV until 10 o'clock and Teacher tells me to sleep. We watch TV together. Teacher asks us which channel we want to see and Teacher helps us to set.

I like to see TV, to sleep, to go to bakery class, to dance, and to sing Karaoke. I am happy today; Teacher bought me cookies and drinks. Teacher tells me I need to lose weight, to be thinner. I take a walk for exercise.

I like to help the teachers to pull the meal delivery cart. I do not have cellphone; Teachers have."

Notes:

[1] Following the Civil War in China, more than one million people moved to Taiwan between 1945 and 1956. About 600,000 of them were soldiers whose families were in China. Local people call this group of veterans 'old taro'. They had difficulty finding local women to marry, so they married women from a disadvantaged social position, including women with disabilities (UDN City, 2011).

[2] In Taiwanese culture, people 'worship' dead parents/ancestors to pay respect to them, which is seen as an aspect of filial piety.

[3] Those people who moved to Taiwan from China with Chiang's Army were called 'foreign province people', including the second generation born in Taiwan.

Ling's story: moving out and having independent life

Ling

Ling was born in 1985 and she has moved in and out of the institution. Two years ago, supported by a social worker who had worked with Ling for almost 10 years, Ling rented an apartment where she lives alone by herself. She works full-time, pays her rent and daily living costs, makes friends, visits her mother and is aware of her rights; and she makes decisions about what she wants and does not want to do. Ling is now receiving support only from the social worker, once a month; she will be totally independent after the service ends in 2018.

"I am now 32 years old and I am old. If you marry at 30, you are too old to give birth to a baby because it is too risky. I was born in P City. My disability certificate card shows that I am with physical and intellectual disability. I do not feel I am intellectually disabled. My father died 10 years ago. When I was six years old, my parents divorced. I have a brother; he died because of fire accident when he was 10 years old. In my life the most unforgettable is that my parents divorced. My brother was very sad for it because he would rather choose to live with my mother. I have searched for my mother by myself and I found her when I was 30 years old. When she saw me she was blaming my father who did not take good care of me to let me become disabled. I was calm when I saw her. She was not as young as the photo that I see. I have an aunt and she lives in L City and she had been my father's girlfriend. During New Year and Moon Festival

Holiday I go to her place in L City. We use LINE[1] to contact each other. My aunt is an immigrant from Thailand and she loves me.

When I was nine years old, my father sent me to the DAWEI Institution.[2] Before I lived in the institution, I did not go to school. I lived in DAWEI for 13 years. When I completed occupational school, I was 22 years old, I wanted to leave DAWEI for a paid job. But the social worker and occupational staff of DAWEI were slow to help me. I went almost crazy having to live in DAWEI after graduation. I know Hope Center through a visit, which was arranged by the junior high school. I called 104 [telephone operational service] to get the phone number of Hope Center. I told the social worker who answered my telephone from Hope that I wanted to work and to have a place to live; at that time I was 21. When I was 22, I moved to the Cherry Community Home[3] where four persons share an apartment. I lived in Cherry for eight years. Now I live alone in an apartment for two years. I chose this apartment and pay for rent by myself. Two years ago, Wei, a social worker of Hope, asked me whether I wanted to move out to live independently. Now I feel very free that I have my own place and I do not need to share it with other people. The downside is that I do not have roommates to share housework. Wei also asked one of roommates whether she also wants to move out to live alone. But her mother does not agree. For me, I do not have parents; I can make decision by myself. I get a rent subsidy from the government. I am happy for my current rented apartment.

I can decide whether I want to cook or not. There is a staff member from Hope Center coming to teach me how to cook, once every two weeks. I prepare food and a recipe and she teaches me how to cook. I have a rabbit; he is my baby. He is now two years old. You can know my rabbit's name from my Facebook.

I like to go shopping, and to play Facebook. I do not like to go out. I do chores work on Saturday. On Sunday I go to church. I buy clothes and manage money by myself.

I drive a scooter to the workplace. It takes 20–25 minutes. I bought the scooter with my savings. I work at a restaurant and I do cleaning work there for eight years since I was 23 years old.

I have two neighbours; we three persons share the house, two floors. I live in the second floor. They are nice to me and we talk and they know me. I have friends from the workplace but we have never gone out together. Some 'teachers' from DAWEI Institution are my friends. Sometimes we go out together.

The most difficult to forget is that I wanted to go to study at the university but the teachers from the occupational school and the Institution were against it. I was very angry that they did not agree. They said that I even could not find a job. Wei is the most influential person in my life. I know her for 10 years. She was accompanying me to take scooter driving licence and to buy the scooter.

I have joined the CRPD meeting that is for young adults with intellectual disabilities.[4] It is once a month, from March to September. I have been there 10 times. We took train from here to Taipei and I went with another young adult. We have 20 persons from all the places joining the CRPD meeting. We also need to prepare our report and I am in the group of law and health. I forgot what the content is in the law part. The health part is related to eating, nutrition, health examination, and going to see a doctor when we are sick. If people say that I am with intellectual disabilities, I am angry. Because this is against CRPD value. CRPD is to protect our rights. I am disabled, but I am not intellectually disabled.

I know some persons from the CRPD meeting. I like one young man but I do not know how to talk with him. His parents might be against.

I am going to Hong Kong and Macau in January with the CRPD group. We are going to visit young people in Hong Kong and Macau. We need to save money. Air tickets and accommodations cost 17,000 dollars. I will prepare 30,000 dollars. I have never been abroad and I only have been to Kinmen Island.[5] I am very excited to go and I was the first person who registered. For some young people of the group, their savings are kept by their parents and they need to ask for their parents' permission. They should have made their own decision whether they want to go.

I am satisfied with my current life. I gave 90 points. Another 10 points would be to have a boyfriend. My current friends are all women. All men whom I like have girlfriends. I have told Wei I want to have a partner who does not have a disability certificate. Wei says that my requirement is too high. So now I only require the person to have a job. I hope I can have a kid, only one. Because I am already 32 years old, I am too old for pregnancy.

I know friends from Church. I am shy to make boyfriends there; unlike me they are not disabled. My aunt wants to introduce a man from Thailand to me. I have seen his picture. He looks not bad; he is deaf. Because he might be more likely to accept me.

Now I do not lack anything. I give my life quality 100 point. I am looking for company instead of a husband. The most important thing in life is to be healthy. Making money is also important. When you have money, you can buy things that you like."

Notes:

[1] LINE is a freeware app for instant communications on electronic devices such as smartphones, tablets and personal computers.

[2] DAWEI Institution opened in 1989 and is managed by a private charity for 200 residents with disabilities.

[3] Cherry Community Home managed by Hope Center, which is managed by a Catholic Charity, providing daycare and residential care services for people with intellectual disabilities.

[4] This is a CRPD Easy Read Group which was organised by a parental association.

[5] This is a local authority located in the south east of Taiwan Island.

Summary

In Taiwan 90% of people with intellectual disabilities live with family and 10% live in an institution. Only a very small proportion, 450 people, less than 0.5%, live in a Community Home. People like Ling, who lives independently, are very rare. It means that almost everyone is 'placed' in an institution when their family are not available for support and, as a consequence, their life is like Chang's and Jenny's, protected and counting on 'teachers'.

Before 2000, institutional residents with intellectual disabilities were requested to get sterilised. For example, Chang had been already sterilised when he lived in FUGEI before becoming an adult. Ling, being 20 years younger than Chang, has a different experience. She lived in the institution from 1994 to 2007 and was not asked to undergo sterilisation. Sterilisation requests are no longer made. Jenny was sterilised after giving birth to two children, and the sterilisation decision was made by her grandmother. Jenny's example echoes Chou and Lu's study (2011) study, which found that the decision to perform sterilisation surgery is often made by the family of women with intellectual disabilities.

Chang has no family and it could be said that he has been locked in the institution for nearly 50 years of his life since he was 'placed' in a homeless shelter as an infant. His social network includes only his 'teachers' and other residents of the institution.

Jenny was born in the early 1960s and both her father and husband were 'old taro'. Both Jenny and her mother are disabled and both their marriages with veterans were arranged by the grandmother. Jenny's grandmother, like those families who had a daughter with disability, expected that Jenny and her mother could have a family, with a husband becoming their carer.

Ling is a successful example of community living reform. Ling's story of moving in and out of an institution, is like many stories from

Western societies (Johnson and Traustadottir, 2005). The difference is that she was 'placed' in the institution in 1994 when she was just a nine-year-old girl. Unlike in the West where institutions were then closing (Gustavsson, 1996; Braddock et al, 2001), DAWEI institution was only established in 1989.

Ling's life now is very different from Chang and Jenny's institutionalised lives. Ling has paid work and income, her scooter and a rabbit, has autonomy to do what she wants to do including to use her savings for travelling, and has her dream to pursue, to find a boyfriend and become a mother. She joined the CRPD meetings to know about her rights and to make friends. In contrast, Chang and Jenny have no chance to learn about their rights under the CRPD. Instead, they still count on their 'teachers' and their daily lives are protected, not only locked in the institution but also under surveillance by family and 'teachers'. How long will such an institutional life remain for people like Chang and Jenny? When will people be able to assert their rights like Ling? Advocacy for the right to live in the community needs to continue in Taiwan.

References

Braddock, D., Emerson, E., Felce, D. and Stancliffe, R.J. (2001) 'Living circumstances of children and adults with mental retardation or developmental disabilities in the United States, Canada, England and Wales, and Australia', *Mental Retardation and Developmental Disabilities Research Reviews*, 7: 115–21.

Chou, Y.C. (2017) 'Implementation of the right of people with disabilities to live independently and to be included in the community in Taiwan: evaluation of laws, policies and programs according to Article 19 of the Convention on the Rights of Persons with Disabilities (CRPD)', *Community Development Quarterly*, 158: 187–207 [in Chinese].

Chou, Y.C. and Schalock, R.L. (2007) 'Trends in residential policies and services for people with intellectual disabilities in Taiwan', *Journal of Intellectual Disability Research*, 51(2): 135–1.

Chou, Y.C. and Lu, Z. (2011) 'Deciding about sterilisation: perspectives from women with an intellectual disability and their families in Taiwan', *Journal of Intellectual Disability Research*, 55(1): 63–74.

Chou, Y.C. and Kröger, T. (2017) 'Application of the ICF in Taiwan: victory of the medical model?', *Disability & Society*, 32(7): 1043–64.

Chou, Y.C., Haj-Yahia, M.M., Wang, F.T.Y. and Fu, L.Y. (2006) 'Social work in Taiwan: an historical and critical review', *International Social Work*, 49(6): 767–78.

Chou, Y.C., Lin, L.C., Pu, C.Y., Lee, W.P. and Chang, S.C. (2008) 'Outcomes and costs of residential services for adults with intellectual disabilities in Taiwan: a comparative evaluation', *Journal of Applied Research in Intellectual Disabilities*, 21, 114–25.

Department of Social Affairs, MOI (Ministry of Interior) (2002) *Report of the fifth national inspection of disability welfare facilities*, Taipei: MOI.

Dessus, S., Shea, J.D. and Shi, M.S. (1995) *Chinese Taipei: The origins of the economic 'Miracle'*, Paris: OECD.

Gold, T.B. (1986) *State and society in the Taiwan Miracle*, London: M.E. Sharpe.

Gustavsson, A. (1996) 'Reforms and everyday meanings of intellectual disability', in J. Tossebro, A. Gustavsson and G. Dyrendahl (eds) *Intellectual disabilities in the Nordic welfare states: Policies and everyday life*, Norway: Norwegian Academic Press, pp 214–37.

Hsiao, S.H. and C.H. Sun (2000) 'Development of social welfare movement in Taiwan since 1980s: change and continuing', in S.H. Hsiao and K.M. Lin (eds) *Social welfare movement in Taiwan*, Taipei: Chu-liu Publishing Company, pp 33–7 [in Chinese].

Johnson, K. and Traustadottir, R. (2005) (eds) *Deinstitutionalisation and people with intellectual disabilities: In and out of institutions*, London: Jessica Kingsley.

UDN City (2011) *Foreign-provincial older soldiers' sadness*. Available at: http://city.udn.com/53171/4605937#ixzz4wJBTn7K5 [in Chinese].

ELEVEN

Intellectual disability policy and practice in twentieth-century United Kingdom

Simon Jarrett and Jan Walmsley

This chapter attempts an overview of the dense and complex history of intellectual disability in the United Kingdom in the twentieth century. Inevitably much of it focuses on legislation and policy emanating from the dominant Westminster parliament and its civil service apparatus. For the first half of the century, we concentrate on the legislative and policy environment in England and Wales, and for the second, mainly on England. Readers seeking a more detailed account, including of developments in Wales, Scotland and Northern Ireland, are referred to Welshman and Walmsley's *Community Care in Perspective* (2006).

We begin with a summary of late-nineteenth-century changes in thought and perspective that laid the groundwork for the radical measures adopted in the early twentieth century. We then focus on the period from 1904 to 1948, dominated by the Mental Deficiency Act 1913, arising from the 1904 Royal Commission on the Care and Control of the Feeble-Minded. The final part covers the period from 1948 to 2001 and sets out the main developments in learning disability policy before telling the story through the lives of four people whose lives span the period.

The paucity of first-hand life stories in the pre-Second World War period is in marked contrast to their emergence in the latter part of the century. This in itself tells a story of at least one way in which change happened, between the controlling and excluding era of the Mental Deficiency Act and movements towards civil liberty in the latter part of the century.

Changing perceptions in the late-nineteenth and early-twentieth century

Radical changes in perception about 'idiocy' emerged in the latter part of the nineteenth century. A small group of 'idiot asylums' were established across the country from the 1850s. These were charitable institutions aimed more at the children of the middle classes than the poorer masses, and small in scale. However, in 1867 the Metropolitan Poor Act established a Metropolitan Asylums Board and by the 1870s three large 'imbecile asylums' had been established, each housing around 1,000 people, the 'idiot' offspring of the London poor (Thomson, 1998, 12–13). The locus of care was switching decisively from the family to the institution, from charitable initiatives to the state, although there never was a move to total institutionalisation. There was always a mixed economy of care, in which families played a prominent role.

Several factors contributed to these changes in perception. The introduction of universal elementary education in 1870 brought into focus a hitherto unidentified, and statistically significant, cohort of school-age children deemed in need of specialist training and intervention (Thomson, 1998, 15). Rising voter participation through the Reform Acts of 1867 and 1884–85 provoked fears in the middle and upper classes about the aptitude of the feeble-minded to be the active and engaged participants that citizen suffrage demanded. The extension of the franchise to almost universal suffrage in 1918 heightened this class anxiety (Thomson, 1998, 51).

There was also the emergence in the late-nineteenth century, gathering pace in the early twentieth, of the pseudo-science of eugenics, based in part on Darwin's evolutionary theory of natural selection. Eugenic theory argued that the racial stock of the population was at risk of degeneration. It identified the feeble-minded person not just with low intelligence and poor bodily and mental health, but also with crime, poverty and disorder. Psychiatrists like Henry Maudsley proposed the idea of the 'moral imbecile', a sort of imbecile who had some form of rational intelligence but had never acquired the higher stage of moral intelligence. The danger of such people, according to eugenicists, was that they possessed cunning intelligence but with no moral framework to guide their actions (Maudsley, 1886, 243–7). By the early twentieth century, the feeble-minded population was framed as a repository of crime, immorality and amorality. Eugenicists argued that it was the duty of the state to intervene and isolate the mentally deficient in some way. In 1904 a Royal Commission on the Care and Control of the Feeble-Minded was the response.

1904–48: from eugenics to the NHS

The twentieth century did not therefore begin auspiciously for those labelled mentally defective. In its first decade 'mental defectives became defined as the central eugenic threat facing the nation' (Thompson, 1998, 20). The 1904 Commission comprised liberal and conservative politicians, lawyers, charity representatives, doctors and civil servants. The charities were the National Association for the Promotion of the Welfare of the Feeble-Minded and the Charity Organisation Society, the latter a radical voluntary organisation preaching eugenic solutions to the problems of poverty, crime and perceived decline of the 'racial stock' (Thompson, 1998, 23-4).

The Commission's 1908 report recommended a system of specialised institutional care for three broad categories: idiots, imbeciles and the feeble-minded. The imbecility category also included moral imbeciles. The report identified large numbers of the mentally deficient inappropriately placed in prisons and lunatic asylums. While not a full-scale eugenicist document, it identified heredity as the primary cause of mental deficiency and downplayed the significance of environment, training or education (Thomson, 1998, 26–33).

There followed a five-year delay before any legislation was enacted, to the frustration of those most keen to see action taken against the feeble-minded population, in particular the Eugenics Education Society (later the Eugenics Society) and the National Association for the Care of the Feeble-minded. In 1911 the two organisations, supported by sympathetic MPs, held a meeting at Westminster to urge action on the government. The main speaker was Alfred Tredgold, one of the country's leading medical 'experts' on mental deficiency, who summed up the prevailing attitude to mental deficiency. He divided people into just two categories:

> Human beings are divisible into two great groups – the *normal* and the *defective*. The normal range from great brilliance to dullness. The defective group … is divided into three degrees, namely *idiocy*, *imbecility* and *feeble-mindedness*. (Anon, 1912, 355; emphasis in original)

Tredgold added that:

> 'All … we desire to do is secure control over those persons whose condition or surroundings are such that their liberty is a source of injury or misery to themselves or a menace to the welfare of the community.' (Anon, 1912, 355–6)

The evening ended with a clarion call to do something towards 'stemming the increasing tide of degeneracy' (Anon, 1912, 357).

Faced with this pressure, within two years the Liberal government introduced an Act to parliament that was overwhelmingly passed. It provided 'an apparatus for the compulsory and permanent segregation of the feeble-minded' (Thomson, 1998, 39). The Mental Deficiency Act 1913 introduced a Board of Control to administer all mental health care (Thomson, 1998, 76), centralising as a state function both the detention and surveillance of the mentally deficient population. There were two central planks to the legislation: the establishment of a network of 'colonies' to house the mentally deficient, and the creation of a system of community control and surveillance for those who were not institutionalised. Resistance to the Act in parliament was feeble, amid a strong cross-party consensus. All three main parties, Conservative, Liberal and Labour, were united in their belief that the degenerate population had to be 'dealt with' in some way (Thomson, 1998, 37–46).

A great irony was that implementation of the Act was delayed by the First World War, which broke out the next year. Many thousands of mentally deficient people, deemed dangerous, unproductive and parasitical in 1913, took up valuable and skilled work roles to fill labour shortages caused by men departing for the front. The problem, as the end of the war loomed, was that they would now have to give up those roles as soldiers returned. In 1917 the Central Association for the Care of the Mentally Defective expressed anxiety that

> Large numbers of low-grade, even imbecile defectives, now in remunerative work … will assuredly leave their work when there is any displacement of labour and we are anxious to make plans for their protection and assistance. (TNA NATS 1/727, 1917)

'Protection and assistance' meant detention or supervision, as the Act would now be fully implemented. There was no consideration that those deemed mentally deficient had shown themselves competent to work and posed no threat during the war years.

The Act provided for three forms of 'care, supervision and control'. These were institutional care, guardianship and community supervision. Institutional care would be the preserve of specialist institutions known as 'colonies'. Guardianship would allow a defective to be placed in the care of a guardian with parental powers over them. Community supervision took the form of a network of statutory health visitors, school nurses and social workers, alongside volunteer home visitors from local mental welfare associations, mainly the Central Association for Mental Welfare (Walmsley et al, 1999, 184–5). All came under the organisational gaze of the Board of Control. The system of community monitoring, surveillance and control was as at least as important as the institutional provision, if not more so. By 1939 there were almost 44,000 defectives under statutory supervision or guardianship, with 46,000 in institutions (Walmsley et al, 1999, 186). The numbers illustrate the lengths to which state authorities were prepared to go, and the public support, or at least acquiescence, they enjoyed, in their aim of controlling the defective population.

The case of Mabel Miles

In 1926 Thomas Lancaster, a 23-year-old coal miner from Rotherham, and Mabel Miles, a 27-year-old 'mental defective', applied for a licence to marry. The Rotherham registrar asked the Registrar General for advice, having received a letter from the Board of Control stating that Mabel Miles was a mental defective detained under her mother's guardianship. Under the Mental Deficiency Act the mother had the same powers over Mabel as if she were a child under 14. The Registrar General asked for a copy of the notice of marriage and ordered that no marriage certificate be issued without instruction from his office. After further enquiries it was confirmed by the Board of Control that Mabel had been detained in an institution for mental defectives between 1916 and 1926. After that she had been transferred to the guardianship of her mother, who was opposed to the marriage. Consent for the marriage was refused and no marriage licence was issued. Mabel Miles' story lies in the impersonal archives of the Board of Control. Unlike the more benign era of the late twentieth century where the voice of the person with intellectual disability began to be heard, we never once hear her voice, or the voice of her prospective husband. We can only trace the sinking of her dream of marriage through the impersonal and inhuman force of the Mental Deficiency Act. (TNA RG/48/159, 1926)

In 1914, the year after the enactment of Mental Deficiency Act, an Elementary Education (Defective and Epileptic Children) Act came into force, compelling all local authorities to provide special schools. A 1925 Mental Deficiency Amendment Act allowed greater use of guardianship as an alternative to institutionalisation. The minor Mental Deficiency Act 1927 expanded institutional provision and placed a duty on local authorities to provide some form of training and occupation. Apart from these few – and in the case of the 1925 and 1927 legislation, minor – exceptions, the 1913 Act remained the enduring legislative framework within which mental deficiency was governed and understood until the Mental Health Act of 1959.

Existing asylums and workhouses adapted to specialist use became repositories for the burgeoning population of mentally deficient patients in the inter-war years. Added to these was the new Colony System which proliferated across the country. The Hedley Committee report (1931) described this institutional innovation, based on an entirely different design to the asylum system. Each colony was a small, usually rural, self-contained world. Between 900 and 1,500 people would live in a typical setting, housed in detached 'villas' for up to 60 people, grouped around a central administrative block. This block always formed a barrier between male and female villas, as separation of the sexes to prevent 'breeding' was deemed essential. Children and adults lived separately and there would also be a special villa for 'difficult cases' – those whose behaviours were regarded as needing control. The villas for 'idiots' and for 'difficult cases' would be as far from the hospital approaches as possible, to avoid offence to visitors. Patients slept in multiple rows, closely packed together in large dormitories with little or no space for privacy or the storage of personal possessions.

In abstract terms the colonies were almost idyllically conceived. As well as the villas there were children's schools, workshops for the adults, kitchens, bakery, laundry, recreation hall (seating up to 750 patients and doubling as a chapel), staff quarters, playing fields and a small mortuary. Many colonies had farms with market gardens, stables, poultry, pigs, herds of cows and greenhouses. As well as nurses they employed farm bailiffs, firemen, engineers and, of course, gatekeepers (Hedley, 1931). Most patients worked unpaid in the laundries and workshops or on the farm. In reality the colonies were harsh, joyless environments, with punitive disciplinary regimes, no concession to individuality and rapidly spreading contagious disease in the closely packed wards, as oral histories looking back on the period have revealed (Potts and Fido, 1991).

Daily life in a colony: discipline and punishment

Sally was detained in an English mental deficiency colony under the 1913 Act in 1942, aged 18:

> "I got a bit fed up of being there and I were missing me family. I used to do things to meself, cut meself 'cos I were depressed, being there so long. I used to break pot and slice it (arm and wrist) when I were in that room

where they locked me ... That's why I run off. The police were after me. I went out (on parole) with another girl and while she were in shop, I run away. Well the police went to me brother's house and they said, "We've got a warrant to see if your sister is here." And they went upstairs to bedroom and everywhere and I wasn't there. I took meself back ... Twice I went back by meself. They say if you go back on your own they can't punish you. They did! When I got back, they put me in that room again! They gave me a cold bath, really cold. They used to put me in a pen. A big square thing with wire round. They put me in there all afternoon and it were snowing. And they took me back at night and put me straight back in that room. I think that's where I got me illness, arthritis. Then I was on floors in that room, no bed, just a mattress ... that's all. And you had tin plates and basins. You weren't allowed any knives and forks, just a spoon ... They used to tie me."

Source: Potts and Fido (1991, 61–2).

There were concessions to ordinary life, recreating the outside leisure world of dances and cinema within the colony, although events were strictly supervised, segregated and highly rule-bound. There were even scout groups, including a bugle band, for young adult males as well as boys.

Daily life in a colony: entertainment

"They used to give us Christmas dances and do's ... that were all right but you couldn't mix. Lads had to have it altogether and girls on their own." (Elizabeth, born 1909)

"We used to go dancing. Females at that end and males at this end. Used to go and say, 'Can I have the honour of this dance, please?'" (Henry, born 1924)

The colony scouts played at the dances:

"Used to have dancing. They all come up to you to dance wi' you. Just the Scouts to play ... there used to be a Scout parade. Used to march all round the villas and back to the Scout huts." (Horace, born 1922)

Source: Potts and Fido (1991, 86–9).

There was a widespread consensus across the British ideological spectrum in the first half of the twentieth century that mental deficiency was in some way a problem that needed to be 'fixed'. It came not just from eugenic theory about threats to the racial stock and the degeneration of civilised society, although this of course played a part. There was also a feeling that in heavily industrialised, newly technological, highly urbanised Western societies, people without sufficient brain power were simply unable to cope with the demands of modernity. They needed, it was argued, protective shielding, and were essentially unproductive. This carried a cost – the Hedley Committee report of 1931 was in part initiated by governmental panic about the costs of the colony system – which was often alluded to in commentary on deficiency. In 1930 Julian Huxley, the zoologist, biologist, humanist and eugenicist, wrote:

> What are we going to do? Every defective man, woman and child is a burden. Every defective is an extra body for the nation to feed and clothe, but produces little or nothing in return. Every defective needs care, and immobilises a certain quantum of energy and goodwill which could otherwise be put to good use. (Quoted in Overy, 2010, 93)

His brother, the novelist and commentator Aldous Huxley, satirised the social engineering dreams of eugenicists in his dystopian novel *Brave New World* in 1932. In the 'brave new world' humans are factory-bred in test tubes to produce specified numbers of people at different grades of intelligence, in order to fulfill different social functions. Menial tasks such as lift-operator are carried out by grinning 'Epsilon-Minus Semi-Morons' (Huxley, 1932/2014, 50). It was satire, but it demonstrated how ideas about deficiency were deeply embedded in national consciousness, and unconsciously adopted. The great and good of 'progressive' politics – such as Sidney and Beatrice Webb, H.G. Wells, Marie Stopes and all the major political parties – signed up to the repression, isolation and eventual eradication of mental deficiency (Overy, 2010, 93–135). It was not so much an ideological standpoint as a shared cultural assumption.

So things stood as a new world war broke out in 1939. The Act that had been passed on the eve of the last war appeared now to a large extent fulfilled, as 90,000 defectives found themselves under the controlling gaze of the British state, either in their community or in an institution. Yet as the battle began against the murderous ideology of Nazism, which had locked itself in a fatal embrace with the 'science' of eugenics, the ideas that had inspired the 1913 legislation would come under challenge.

This war would, like its 1914–18 predecessor, see 'useless' mentally deficient people transferred to vital occupations to assist the war effort, while their institutions were commandeered for treatment of the war wounded. In 1945 as the horrors of Nazi genocide against the 'unfit' population came to light, the proponents of eugenics beat a tactical retreat. State-provided long-stay hospitals were brought under the umbrella of the new National Health Service from 1948, while newly emboldened parents began campaigns for the rights of their intellectually disabled sons and daughters. In changing times language changed also – the mentally deficient became the mentally handicapped.

1948–2001: from the National Health Service to *Valuing People*

Developments in the UK after the Second World War mirrored in many respects developments in other countries influenced by the USA. The era of institutions gave way to largely state-provided community care in the later part of the century, influenced by a powerful and vocal parents' movement, followed by a proliferation of providers and fragmentation, under the banner of 'personalisation', and culminating in visionary White Papers, *Valuing People* (Department of Health, 2001) in England and Wales and *The Same as You?* (Scottish Government, 2000) in Scotland.

Immediately following the Second World War, provision of institutional care was taken over by the state via a transfer of local authority, charity and privately run hospitals into the National Health Service in 1948. This confirmed the adoption of a medical model, run by doctors and staffed by nurses and unqualified nursing auxiliaries. Conditions in institutions did not alter markedly. Indeed, the hospitals were starved of resources, and many struggled to recruit staff (Keilty and Woodley, 2013). The leitmotif of services, until the 1970s, and later in some areas, was waiting lists for hospital care, and very limited provision outside.

There was a discernible shift in rhetoric from the late 1940s, although changes on the ground followed much more slowly. A vigorous parents' movement began in 1947, with the founding of the first local Society for the Parents of Mentally Handicapped Children in Cambridge (Shennan, 1980; Rolph, 2002). By the mid-1950s there were over 200 branches, variously lobbying locally for provision outside hospitals, fundraising, and setting up and running nurseries, holiday chalets, clubs and even occupation centres and residential homes (Rolph, 2002). They also lobbied nationally, arguing for every child to have the right to schooling (achieved in 1970 in England), and contributed to the Percy Committee in 1957, which led to the Mental Health Act 1959 (Welshman, 2006). One aim of the parents' movement, in which they were remarkably successful, was to change perceptions of their children from the eugenic menace of the 1930s to a recognition of them as fellow human beings, albeit to be pitied rather than respected as equal citizens (Walmsley, 2000).

In common with most Western countries, from the late 1970s policy was increasingly influenced by normalisation and, later, social role valorisation (see Introduction in this book). Integration, the use of mainstream services, an ordinary life in ordinary streets with a paid job and local community activities became the aspiration from as early as the 1970s (Department of Health and Social Security, 1979). How to achieve this was unclear, but the ideal remained. In Wales a major initiative, the All Wales Strategy of 1983, aimed to secure for people a full life in the community. It was led from central government and, highly unusually, funding was attached (Felce et al, 1998).

Provision of 'community care' – which at the time referred to state-run hostels and day centres – was patchy until after the 1971 White Paper *Better Services for the Mentally Handicapped* (Department of Health and Social Security/Welsh Office, 1971). This was prompted by press exposure of abuse in Ely Hospital, Cardiff, which brought to public attention appalling conditions in mental handicap hospitals: overcrowded, under-staffed and hidden from scrutiny (Morris, 1969; Donges, 1982). The White Paper, while not committing to hospital closure, did acknowledge that it was a system unsuitable for many housed within it. Targets were set for local authorities to open day and residential provision, and, while as ever progress was slower than hoped, a boost was given to developments in most areas (Walmsley, 2006a). Initially, influenced by a Mencap-funded experiment in Slough, the community care ideal was a large hostel situated near a training centre (Walmsley, 2006b). Over time smaller group homes were favoured, and by the end of the century the ideal was independent living in own house or flat. In practice, the majority of people continued to live with their families as there was never sufficient provision, and some families preferred this (Emerson and Hatton, 2015). Nor had institutions totally disappeared.

It is difficult to pinpoint the precise date when it became policy to close all hospitals (Ingham, 2012), but by the 1980s this was the direction of travel. Progress was slow – the last NHS hospital did not officially close until 2010, and many smaller NHS campuses, such as that at Calderstones, Lancashire, remained open for long after that date. But deinstitutionalisation, heavily influenced by Wolf Wolfensberger's vision of social role valorisation – was the principal policy shift of the 1980s and 1990s (Ingham, 2012).

At the same time, ideas coming from the wider disability movement, about independent living, and personal assistance under the direct control of disabled people, made inroads into official thinking (Walmsley, 2006b). Direct payments became an option from 1997, and the 2001 White Paper, *Valuing People*, made 'Independence, Choice, Rights and Inclusion' its central principles (Department of Health, 2001). Social inclusion, the use of those services and facilities that everyone uses, became the mantra, with segregated specialist services seen as the enemy, paving the way for the closure of those day centres earlier generations had fought for. Welshman and Walmsley describe this as 'the zenith of a period of optimism swelling with possibilities and promises of a better life for this most disadvantaged of groups' (2006, 2). In the early twenty-first century, pilots demonstrated that giving the budget to a person with a learning disability opened the way for them to make choices, and live an ordinary life (Needham and Glasby, 2014), and thus was the preference for individualised packages of care born (Walmsley, 2006b).

The rest of the chapter is devoted to the stories of three people, two of whom were interviewed by the second author in 1991, the third, one of England's most celebrated campaigners.

Life stories: Beryl, Bert and Mabel

Beryl: a life lived at home

'Beryl' was born in 1932. Her story is of a woman whose life was lived initially with family and latterly with the scaffolding of the type of 'community care' characteristic of the late twentieth century, including a full-time placement at a training centre.

Beryl recalled her childhood:

> "Learnt meself to walk, walking along the furniture and all that, yeh ....
> Didn't really do nothing till I was 7 years old ... I had lessons at home ....
> I didn't used to go out, weren't no centres then." (Interview with author, 1991[1])

Beryl's testimony refers to the fact that where she lived, the only non-institutional provision until the mid-1950s was small 'occupation centres' for children and teenagers, and until large centres opened late in the 1950s, there was nothing, other than home tutoring.

Beryl lived with her parents into adulthood. She became a carer for her mother after her father died. When her mother too died, Beryl's brother who, in her words, 'kept an eye' on her, got her a flat and a place at the new adult training centre in 1966. At the time of our interview (1993), Beryl was still at this centre, and was looking forward, with some trepidation, to 'retirement', as she termed it. She had done contract work at the centre for most of her time there, but, as was the fashion at the time, this had been phased out in favour of 'social education'. Beryl was dismissive:

> "We ain't got nothing .... Nothing, we an't got none work for months and months. Years ago we got all sorts of work. I don't need to learn cooking really, what good gardening, I ain't got a garden, even when I were younger I didn't do it."

Beryl sums up in one pithy paragraph the history of day centres in the mid-twentieth century, and her story illustrates the impact the development of services had on her life. My impression from meeting her and two friends was that she was significant in supporting her friends to manage independently. They lived in nearby flats, attended the centre and were frequently organised and fed by Beryl.

Beryl did not have a partner. When asked about boyfriends Beryl's response was terse:

> "No, don't want one."

Had she imbibed the eugenic philosophy, that people like her must not get involved with men? This had not entirely changed even by the 1990s. Beryl told me that at the centre "they stop it a little bit. One girl she got sent to Silsoe so she lost her boyfriend."

Beryl was robustly self-sufficient and independent. Deprived by circumstance of conventional adult roles she had built a life revolving around supporting her friends with wry observations about life at the centre.

Note: [1] All quotations are taken from Walmsley (1995, ch 7).

Bert: a life lived in institutional care[1]

Bert's story is illustrative of the young working-class men who got into trouble with the law and found themselves in the mental handicap[2] system. Bert was born in the 1940s and was in Bromham, a mental handicap hospital, when interviewed in 1991.

> "I didn't go to school, didn't go to school till I was 6 and I wouldn't learn, they sent me to a backward school but I never used to go … All me mates that was brainy they did National Service,[3] all me mates that were at school with me."

Bert's great regret was that he had not been able to join the army, unlike his father and brother. He had trained as a plumber but could not pass his apprenticeship because he could not read. Then he got a job as a hod carrier on the buildings. That did not last and he then committed a minor crime. This is what he said:

> "I went to Leavesden[4] first time, though when I got in a bit of trouble. I think it was a factory break-in somebody shopped us, I got taken a year, I did 6 months then I ran away, got a job on the buildings, then a second time I got in trouble again, I went to Magistrates, they said we can't send you there (to Leavesden) cos you run away, you kept outa trouble we coulda discharged you, got sent to Magull[5] for 6 years. I came straight from Magull to here. They said you done your time, and you've lost your mother we'll send you to Bromham you know."

He was still there, having spent almost all his adult life being punished for a crime. Of Magull, he said:

> "Hard life, I've had a hard life … well they used to boot them, put them in a straitjacket and boot them … but I was told Rampton[6] was worse."

The course of his life had been heavily influenced by his mother's death. This, he believed, was the reason he had not been sent home after his sentence. He cried when remembering that he had not been allowed out to go to the funeral.

> "The chief wouldn't let me go there, the chief what belonged to the hospital. I was bad for a week though, when mum died. I was upset. I hadn't seen her since she was alive, since I was at home."

Bert was, when I met him, expecting to leave the hospital, which was already running down in preparation for closure in 1996. His brother Don was a plumber and he was hoping to get a job with him. In the meantime he spent his days working on the hospital site, collecting laundry and running errands as a deputy porter. Unpaid.

He did not deny having romantic inclinations. He told me of a girlfriend whom he had met on a holiday. But she was in an institution 200 kilometres away. Meeting was not an option. They exchanged letters instead.

Notes:

[1] See Walmsley, 1995, ch 7 for all quotes in this box.

[2] 'Mental handicap' was the official term 1971–c.1990.

[3] All youths had to spend two years in the army unless exempt on health grounds.

[4] Leavesden was a large mental handicap hospital on the edge of London.

[5] One of three 'special hospitals' for the criminally insane.

[6] Another 'special hospital'.

Mabel Cooper, 1944–2013: a life of campaigning

Mabel was a well-known self-advocate, having published, with Dorothy Atkinson, several versions of her life story (Cooper, 1997; Atkinson and Cooper, 2000; Cooper with Atkinson, n.d.). She uncovered the story of her early life through accessing her case notes, when she was in her fifties. They showed that her mother had been begging in London with Mabel as a baby, having been thrown out by her father, who disapproved of her choice of husband. She was labelled 'feeble-minded' and taken to Darenth Park,[1] and put in a succession of children's homes, and then, aged 13, in St Lawrence's Hospital,[2] where she remained for 20 years. She was selectively mute in St Lawrence's, only saying 'yes' or 'no'. She graphically described conditions in the hospital:

> You think you were going into a madhouse .... You could hear people screaming and shouting inside. (Cooper with Atkinson, n.d., 13)

> There was bars on the windows, it was just like a prison ... you didn't have toys, no toys whatsoever ... There was no school there, they only let you use your hands by making baskets ... That's all you did Because in them days they said you wasn't capable of doing anything else. (Cooper with Atkinson, n.d., 14)

Mabel was finally released from St Lawrence's in around 1975, initially to a 50-bedded hostel for women.

> This was the same as St Lawrence's, the only difference was it was a house. (Cooper with Atkinson, n.d., 24)

She was taken back to the hospital to spend the day there. With help from Eva, a nurse she had befriended in the hospital, Mabel left the hostel, and lived in various places, each time with more autonomy. In her autobiography she describes graphically the experience of coming out of institutions:

> I thought the children were midgets ... I never saw children, only children in wheelchairs ... not children running about and doing all the things they are doing ... I'd never been on a bus or a train. Because you never went. These were the things you didn't do. (Cooper with Atkinson, n.d., 26)

Mabel went on to become Chair of London People First, then the largest self-advocacy organisation in the UK, and then joined the Open University's Social History of Learning Disability Research Group of which she was an active member for the rest of her life. Her achievements and contributions to the University were recognised in 2010, when she was awarded an Honorary Degree.

Mabel believed passionately that the way to change attitudes was to influence young children. She spent her latter years going into schools in London to tell her life story, supported by her friend and advocate Jane Abraham.

Mabel's story illustrates the resilience shown by many former residents of institutions, and the opportunities open to a talented woman with learning disabilities in the late twentieth century. A film was made of her life, to carry on the work she started with schools.[3]

Notes:

[1] A large mental handicap hospital on the edge of London.

[2] Another mental handicap hospital on the edge of London.

[3] No Longer Shut Up, available on YouTube.

Conclusion

The story of intellectual disability in the UK in the twentieth century mirrors other English-speaking countries. The century began with a loud clamour about a eugenic threat and a consensus that segregation in institutions was the answer. Although only about half of those 'ascertained' as defective actually lived in institutions, they were seen as the ideal. Many lives were blighted by this myopia. This certainty slowly gave way under pressure from families, scandals and new ideas such as normalisation. The pace of change in the last quarter of the century accelerated, institutions were discredited and various types of 'community care' were adopted, moving from a preference for large hostels and segregated day centres to an emphasis on integration or inclusion, use of mainstream services, small homes, independent living, and, at the very end of the century, a budget to enable people to buy their own assistance. It may be these developments that led historians McDonagh, Goodey and Stainton to describe the UK as one of the countries that has taken deinstitutionalisation furthest (2018, 22). At the time, the present authors recall, it did seem the start of a new and wonderful era, hard to remember at the time of writing (2018) when a combination of public funding austerity, diminishing social care and welfare budgets, uncontrolled marketisation and the unfettered operation of large and hard-to-restrain private providers of 'specialist' care led the United Nations to state that the UK was failing to uphold the UN Convention on the Rights of Persons with Disabilities (UN Committee on the Rights of Persons with Disabilities, 2016). A consortium of UK disability groups stated that 'the Government will claim we're world leaders in disability rights, but actually, things have gone rapidly backwards in the last ten years' (Bulman, 2017). The high hopes associated with the *Valuing People* (Department of Health, 2001) and *The Same as You?* (Scottish Government, 2000) White Papers seem in 2018 under real threat.

References

Anon (1912) 'The Feeble-minded Control Bill: House of Commons meeting, December 5th, 1911', *The Eugenics Review*, Vol III, 355–8.

Atkinson, D. and Cooper, M. (2000) 'Parallel stories' in L. Brigham, D. Atkinson, M. Jackson, S. Rolph and J. Walmsley (eds) *Crossing boundaries: Change and continuity in the history of learning disabilities*, Kidderminster: British Institute of Learning Disabilities, pp 15–26.

Bulman, M. (2017) 'Government accused of breaching UN convention in its treatment of disabled people', *The Independent*, 21 August.

Cooper, M. (1997) 'Mabel Cooper's life story', in D. Atkinson, M. Jackson and J. Walmsley, *Forgotten lives: Exploring the history of learning disability*, Kidderminster: BILD.

Cooper M with Atkinson D (undated) *I'd like to know why*, private publication.

Department of Health and Social Security/Welsh Office (1971) *Better Services for the Mentally Handicapped*, Cmnd 4683, London: HMSO.

Department of Health and Social Security (1979) *Report of the Committee of Inquiry into Mental Handicap, Nursing and Care* [the Jay Report], London: The Stationery Office.

Department of Health (2001) *Valuing People: A New Strategy for Learning Disability for the 21st Century*, Norwich, The Stationery Office.

Donges, G. (1982) *Policy making for the mentally handicapped*, Aldershot: Gower.

Emerson, E., Hatton, C. et al (2015) *People with learning disabilities in England 2015: Services and supports,* Improving Health and Lives: Learning Disability Observatory, Department of Health. Available at: https://www.gov.uk/government/uploads/system/uploads/attachment_data/file/613182/PWLDIE_2015_main_report_NB090517.pdf

Felce, D., Grant, G. et al (1998) *Towards a full life: Researching policy innovation for people with learning disabilities*, London: Butterworth Heinemann.

Hedley, W. (1931) *Report of the Departmental Committee on Colonies for Mental Defectives* [the Hedley Report], London: HMSO.

Huxley, A. (1932/2014) *Brave new world*, London: Vintage.

Ingham, N. (2012) 'Organisational change and resistance: an oral history of the rundown of a long stay institution for people with learning disabilities', Unpublished PhD thesis, Milton Keynes: Open University.

Keilty, T. and Woodley, K. (2013) *No going back*, Sheffield: Centre for Welfare Reform.

Maudsley, H. (1883) *Body and Will*, London: Kegan Paul Trench.

McDonagh, P., Goodey, C.F. and Stainton, T. (eds) (2018) *Intellectual disability: A conceptual history, 1200–1900*, Manchester: Manchester University Press.

Morris, P. (1969) *Put away*, London: Routledge Kegan Paul.

Needham, C. and Glasby, J. (eds) (2014) *Debates in personalisation*, Bristol: Policy Press.

Overy, R. (2010) *The morbid age: Britain and the crisis of civilization*, London, Penguin.

Potts, M. and Fido, R. (1991) *'A fit person to be removed': Personal accounts of life in a mental deficiency institution*, Plymouth: Northcote House.

Rolph, S. (2002) *Reclaiming the past*, Milton Keynes: Open University.

Scottish Government (2000) *The Same As You*. Available at: https://www2.gov.scot/resource/doc/1095/0001661.pdf (accessed 10 January 2019).

Shennan, V. (1980) *Our Concern: The story of the National Association for Mentally Handicapped Children and Adults*, London: National Association for Mentally Handicapped Children and Adults.

Thomson, M. (1998) *The problem of mental deficiency: Eugenics, democracy, and social policy, c. 1870–1959*, Oxford: Clarendon Press.

UN Committee on the Rights of Persons with Disabilities (2016) *Inquiry concerning the United Kingdom of Great Britain and Northern Ireland carried out by the Committee under article 6 of the Optional Protocol to the Convention Report of the Committee*, New York: United Nations. Available at: www.ohchr.org/EN/HRBodies/CRPD/Pages/InquiryProcedure.aspx (accessed 21 December 2017).

Walmsley, J. (1995) *Gender, caring and learning disability*, Milton Keynes: Open University.

Walmsley, J., Atkinson, D. and Rolph, S. (1999) 'Community care and mental deficiency 1913 to 1945' in P. Bartlett and D. Wright (eds) *Outside the walls of the asylum: The history of care in the community 1750–2000*, London: Athlone Press.

Walmsley, J. (2000) 'Straddling boundaries: the changing role of voluntary organisations' in D. Atkinson et al (eds) *Crossing boundaries: Continuity and change in the history of learning disabilities*, Kidderminster: BILD.

Walmsley, J. (2006a) 'Organisations and structures, 1971–2001' in J. Welshman and J. Walmsley (eds) *Community care in perspective: Care, control and citizenship*, London: MacMillan.

Walmsley, J. (2006b) 'Ideology, ideas and care in the community, 1971–2001' in J. Welshman and J. Walmsley (eds) *Community care in perspective: Care, control and citizenship*, London: MacMillan.

Welshman, J. (2006) 'Ideology, ideas and care in the community, 1948–71' in J. Welshman and J. Walmsley (eds) *Community care in perspective: Care, control and citizenship*, London: MacMillan.

Welshman, J. and Walmsley, J. (eds) (2006) *Community care in perspective: Care, control and citizenship*, London: MacMillan.

Archival material

The National Archives:

TNA NATS 1/727 (1917) *Central Association for the care of the mentally defective: request for information regarding rejection of soldiers for mental deficiency 1917–18*.

TNA RG/48/159 (1926) *Proposed marriage of adult mental defective*.

TWELVE

From social menace to unfulfilled promise: the evolution of policy and practice towards people with intellectual disabilities in the United States

Philip M. Ferguson

Centuries (as well as decades and years) are malleable demarcations of time. Held to a literal calendar, the 100-year periods are rigid divisions, changing over on the 'double zero' years. Yet most people experience centuries as eras organised around key events, dramatic discoveries or major social and economic shifts. Also implied with this constructivist approach to the periodisation of history is that centuries differ from group to group, from setting to setting. Sometimes we recognise these beginnings and endings in the moment. Most Americans, I would argue, think of the twenty-first century as beginning not on 1 January 2000, but on 11 September 2001, with the indelible images of planes flying into the World Trade Center in New York City. That is when and how we came to think of our place in the world, both individually and as a nation, in radically different ways. Many historians would agree that the founding fathers of America (George Washington, Thomas Jefferson and so on) knew at the time of their actions in declaring independence from England, that it was the beginning of a radically new era. To give any coherence to an overview of the nineteenth century in the United States, then, you almost have to have it begin in 1789 or even 1776, rather than the calendar date of 1800. However, sometimes these century markers are known only with hindsight and remain open to dispute. The evolution of events gains temporal meaning only in retrospect, with some groups finding importance in one key event, while others find significance in another.

This chapter uses contemporaneous accounts and retrospective interpretations to argue that the history of intellectual disability in the USA in the twentieth century can be experientially understood to run from around 1908 to around 1999. These dates reflect the introduction and rapid spread of the Binet intelligence test at the beginning (Zenderland, 1998) and the landmark Supreme Court case, *Olmstead v. L.C.*, 527 U.S. 581 (1999), establishing a right to community-based living (with some key deference given to professional judgement) for individuals with intellectual disabilities at the end. A further division into three separate eras can help to shape our understanding of how circumstances in the USA for individuals with intellectual disabilities have simultaneously undergone dramatic change and remained frustratingly the same. I broadly categorise these as: the eugenics era; the rise of family advocacy; and the rise of self-advocacy. For each of the three periods within this constructed twentieth century, a brief narrative of an individual from that era is provided to ground the analysis in the actual lives of actual people. Each narrative is then followed with a short analysis of the themes that emerge from the individual stories.

Segregation and surgery: Deborah Kallikak and the eugenics era

Emma's story

Deborah Kallikak was a star, at least within certain circles of professionals who ran institutions and special education programmes for the so-called feeble-minded population in the first decades of the twentieth century. Emma Wolverton, on the other hand, was unknown to most. They were, in fact, the same person. Deborah Kallikak was the fictitious name created by the psychologist Henry Goddard for his influential account of Deborah and her relatives (Goddard, 1912) that became the best known of the 'family histories' about supposed generations of defective families being published at the time (Rafter, 1988). These 'studies' were used to justify eugenic efforts to control the 'social menace' of feeble-mindedness through segregation and sterilisation, by supposedly documenting how intellectual deficits were passed down through generations. Deborah Kallikak and her relatives became Goddard's best example of inherited deficit.

Emma Wolverton, on the other hand was left unnamed and unrecognised to all but those at the institution where she lived out her life. Emma, not Deborah, was the flesh-and-blood person sent to the institution in New Jersey aged eight. Emma, not Deborah, was kept at the institution until her death in 1978 aged 89 (Smith and Wehmeyer, 2012, 214). It was Emma who liked cats; enjoyed writing letters; played instruments and read music. It was Emma who could read and write by the age of 10; who made some of her own clothing; who was chosen to serve as a teacher's aide for the institution kindergarten. It was Emma who knew that Goddard had written a book about her, a fact she wore as a badge of honour within the confines of the institution (Reeves, 1938). The image of Deborah manufactured by Goddard to suit his argument for identification and segregation of his newly named category of 'morons' was wrong in its details and fictionalised in its portrayal (Smith and Wehmeyer, 2012).

Emma's real name was not widely known until after her death (Straney, 1994). Only in the past decade has the life story of the real Emma Wolverton come to replace the myth of Deborah Kallikak. As two of the scholars most responsible for that rediscovery have put it: '*Her* name was Emma, not Deborah. Emma Wolverton. *We* at least owe her the respect of calling her by her name' (Smith and Wehmeyer, 2012, 216).

Themes and analysis

Goddard did more than popularise the myth of the Kallikak family. He was also one of the key individuals in popularising the Binet IQ test in the USA as the tool best suited to identifying and classifying people like Emma Wolverton with a speed and efficiency previously unknown (Zenderland, 1998). In 1908, Goddard (or perhaps his assistant, Elizabeth Kite) translated part of Binet's test from French (Goddard, 1911). Over the next two years, Goddard and others (Kuhlmann, 1911) successfully put forth the new test as a powerful yet simple way of psychologically assessing individuals with a precision and certainty previously unavailable. The promulgation of the IQ test enabled professionals like Goddard to create an entirely new category of mild intellectual disability: the 'moron' (formed from the Greek for 'fool') who was otherwise hard to tell from the merely 'backward' child. The test in turn greatly enhanced the ability of educators and psychologists to identify children supposedly suitable for the rapidly expanding special education classrooms and schools. The challenge at the beginning of the twentieth century, then, became to identify as rapidly as possible as many people as possible for control and segregation from the general population. The name of science was used to justify the policy of social Darwinism, where the menace of the feeble-minded was paramount and prevention the only salvation.

This obsession with professional control and custody of individuals identified as idiots, imbeciles or morons led to the dramatic expansion of institutions, (often called state schools or asylums). In 1906, a special census found some 15,318 housed in 42 public and private asylums. Combined with those in so-called 'insane asylums', the number of individuals identified as having intellectual or psychiatric disabilities totalled some 164,498 (United States Census Bureau,1906). By 1940, the Census found (not counting children under 14), an increase to almost 600,000 (US Census, 1943, p. 6).

In addition to the expansion of large institutions as custodial facilities for 'mentally deficient' populations, the first decades of the twentieth century also saw the rapid growth of special educational schools and classrooms in urban districts throughout the country. While educational rhetoric and intention often cited the pedagogical benefits of these self-contained settings for 'backward' or 'deficient' children, there was also an underlying motive of social control similar to the impetus for asylums (Osgood, 2008). The rapid adoption of the Binet test allowed, for the first time, an efficient and seemingly objective method for identifying thousands of children seen as inappropriate for the regular classroom. It was acknowledged by one leading educator as 'the chief stimulus' for the expansion of separate classrooms (Wallin, 1924, 41) with 'hundreds of thousands' of tests administered annually (Osgood, 2008, 47). A 1928 survey found a total of 51,814 'subnormal and backward' children in some 218 school systems across 33 states (Davies, 1930, 299).

However, segregation was only one strategy for control and prevention of more generations of Kallikaks. The other means proposed by the psychologists and other so-called 'progressives' of the era was the involuntary sterilisation of feeble-minded people. Between 1907, when the first sterilisation law was enacted in Indiana, and 1941, some 38,087 'defectives' were sterilised (Reilly, 1991), sometimes with the supposed consent of parents or other family members, but often on the sole authority of the state. Through segregation or surgery, the goal for the first decades of the twentieth century was to control, if not prevent, the 'menace' of feeble-mindedness from further debilitating mainstream society.

Out of the shadows: Rosemary Kennedy and the rise of family advocacy

Rosemary's story

At first glance, Emma Wolverton and Rosemary Kennedy seem very different individuals. Emma was born in poverty and institutionalised at an early age. Rosemary was born to a family of growing wealth and power and lived largely with her parents until adulthood. Emma was a subject of public scrutiny, albeit under a name given to her without her permission or request. Rosemary was a 'hidden' or 'missing' Kennedy (Larson, 2015; Koehler-Pentacoff; 2016), even though much of her childhood was spent in the public attention shared with her brothers and sisters. Yet, despite these important differences, Emma and Rosemary both have stories whose circumstances symbolise their separate eras. Emma, in her imposed Kallikak persona, personified the 'dangers' of uncontrolled and unprevented feeble-mindedness, her story reflecting the involuntary stigmatisation and custodial segregation that symbolised the early decades of the twentieth century. Rosemary's role in the context of her powerful family becomes symbolic of her era, a transition narrative from hiddenness to visibility; from family shame and subjection to family advocacy and activism.

Rosemary Kennedy was born on 13 September 1918, the third of nine children. Her older brother, John, would become President of the United States in 1961. Rosemary had a difficult birth and it was not long before her mother, Rose Kennedy, noticed delays in language development and motor skills (Koehler-Pentacoff, 2016). Judged unsuccessful in several public schools, Rosemary was educated at home by private tutors until the age of 16. Despite being assessed, aged seven, as mentally deficient by a Harvard psychologist, neither parent would acknowledge the label. Like many parents in the 1920s and 1930s, they were told to institutionalise their child. However, having the financial resources to resist, they kept Rosemary at home throughout most of her childhood.

In 1941, at the age of 23, Rosemary underwent an unproven and controversial procedure known as pre-frontal lobotomy (Larson, 2015). As with many of these procedures, despite the professionals' promises of cure or amelioration, the operation on Rosemary left her much more significantly disabled, physically and intellectually. She was institutionalised in 1949 at a private facility in Wisconsin and stayed there until her death in 2005. Her father never saw Rosemary again after the surgery. Her mother did not see her for 20 years. Her brothers and sisters were told only that her 'behaviour' had worsened and she had been sent to a facility that could control her. They were told she was to have no visitors.

Only in the 1960s, with the campaign and election of John Kennedy as President, did Rosemary's story begin to be told. While her parents never escaped their generation's assumption of shame and silence about having a 'defective' child, the siblings became, to varying degrees, public advocates on behalf of intellectually disabled people and their families. Eunice Kennedy, Rosemary's younger sister, pushed her brother, the President, to shine the light of public policy and social awareness on a population that had, heretofore, been left in the shadows (Shorter, 2000). Robert Kennedy, as Senator from the State of New York, would make several public visits to overcrowded institutions, the press and photographers in tow, to expose the cruel abuse and neglect occurring in the nation's human warehouses.

Themes and analysis

The years from about 1940 to about 1970 constituted a complicated mixture of old attitudes and new reforms. At first, as we have seen with the story of Rosemary Kennedy, even disabled children from wealthy families were often hidden and invisible. Professionals often considered parents as much of a problem as the child with disabilities (Ferguson, 2008). By the end of the era, early parent activism and cohesion into a national advocacy group were transforming how society viewed intellectual disability. However, even with the rise of parent activism and public attention, the person with disability remained largely voiceless. The transition was benevolent but patronising; from social menace to innocent child. Parent advocacy brought their children out of the shadows, only to argue that an improved and better funded institution or segregated school was the appropriate goal for social reform. This contradiction left parents proclaiming the rights for their children as tragic victims rather than moral dangers, but who, in either case, must be sheltered and secured for life. As one historian has put it: 'parents created a needs-based narrative depicting their offspring as "eternal children" and a human-rights narrative stressing the obligation of the state to provide for its members, regardless of their abilities' (Carey, 2009, 105).

In 1950, the first national advocacy organisation dedicated to the support of intellectually disabled persons and their families was started as a coalition of some 23 local parent groups that had sprung up around the country. By 1958, the National Association for Retarded Children had grown to some 550 local chapters (Trent, 1994, 241). The 1950s also saw the beginning of what was to become a distinct genre of writing: the parent memoir. At first these were written by celebrities such as the writer Pearl Buck (Buck, 1950) or Dale Evans Rogers (Rogers, 1953) the country and western television star (together with her husband Roy Rogers). Soon, they became more common, if still not ever truly representative of the entire population of families of disabled children.

By the end of this era in the 1960s, the parent movement was fully entrenched and claimed the members of the Kennedy family as part of their group. New policy initiatives began. Criticism of professionals became acceptable in an unprecedented way. Still, the discontent was emerging that the portrayal of intellectually disabled adults as 'eternal children' was silencing with a velvet glove those who previously been stilled with the hammer of state control. The era of self-advocacy and full participation was still to come.

Promises made but unfulfilled: Ian Ferguson and the rise of self-advocacy

Ian's story

Ian Ferguson was born in 1969. Soon after birth he developed complications from surgery that left him with a variety of intellectual and physical disabilities. He uses a wheelchair and has a laundry list of labels (cerebral palsy, significant intellectual disability, vision and speech impairments) that make him eligible for various programmes designed for his support. He also has a warped sense of humour, an ability to communicate very clearly using behaviour rather than words, and an enjoyment of music that he is happy to share with others. None of these latter qualities make him eligible for any programmes, but they have become the central part of what makes him the individual that others in his life know and love.

Ian is now 49 years old. His story is a convenient exemplar of a generation of people with disabilities who came of age in the 1970s and 1980s in the USA. When Ian was five years old in 1974, state law where he lived excluded him from attending public school. Along with almost one million other young people with disabilities, he was deemed 'too severe' or 'too challenging' to benefit from public school. One year later, the federal government passed what is now called the Individuals with Disabilities Education Act, guaranteeing for the first time that Ian and every other child, regardless of degree or type of disability, could have what the law called 'a free and appropriate public education'. That law was the first of many in this period that would create legal rights and protections for Ian and his generation. By 1990, the Americans with Disabilities Act extended protections for Ian into adulthood. 'Accessibility' and 'reasonable accommodations' became the era's bywords.

As with many in Ian's generation, his life is demonstrably better than it would have been had he been born 30 or 40 years earlier. There is no public institution for people with intellectual disabilities in his state. While employment is not mandated as a legal right, Ian has a part-time job doing real work, for real pay, in an integrated college campus setting. He lives in his own home, with a combination of federal and state dollars supporting the personal assistants that make that possible.

It is, in short, a life full of friends, family and community inclusion bolstered by an array of programmes that both benefit and protect him. Still, frustrations remain, and others of his generation are still waiting for the same benefits.

Themes and analysis

The record of change in US society over the last three decades of the twentieth century (and into the twenty-first) has been dramatic for many minority groups. There have been prominent advances in civil rights for women and racial minorities. Other groups laid the groundwork for increased recognition and acceptance that truly gained traction in the last decade. Not the least of these groups is the disability community in general, and the intellectual disability community in particular. The advances cut across the domains of life, involving legislation, judicial decisions and theoretical reformulations that, taken together, have truly shifted the country's thinking about intellectually disabled individuals. At the same time, the undeniable advances have also served to raise expectations about how far we still have to go.

Philosophically, this period saw a dramatic change in the assumptions both about the rights and capacities of people with disabilities, and about the concept of disability itself. Following the lead of the Civil Rights Movement and the Women's Liberation Movement, the 1970s disability community began to demand their own voices be heard. The 'People First' movement was one of the earliest self-advocacy groups demanding visibility and attention for people with intellectual disabilities (Carey, 2009, 254–8). An academic branch of the disability rights movement started to challenge the very concept of 'disability', arguing that the meaning of 'disability' itself was more socially constructed than medically discovered. A new framework for the policy and practice of supporting intellectually disabled people, first called 'normalisation' and later 'social role valorisation', challenged the symbolism of diminishment and infantilisation hidden in traditional arrangements for people with intellectual disabilities (Wolfensberger, 1972). In short, in a few brief years, the conversation about disabled people changed dramatically. Those who for centuries had been treated as voiceless burdens, when noticed at all, were now asserting their rights to be seen and heard, granted their place in the community, and accepted as productive and contributing citizens.

In legal terms, Ian's generation was the first to be guaranteed access to public education, in what the law described as 'the least restrictive environment' possible. Signed into law in 1975, the legislation has shown both the promise and the failure of reform efforts. While the law guarantees access to public education, for many students with intellectual disabilities that education remains largely segregated from their non-disabled peers. In 1990, the Americans with Disabilities Act (ADA) promised to be the 'civil rights Act' for the disability community. In many ways, the United Nations Convention on the Rights of People with Disabilities (CRPD) borrows some of its themes and language (employment rights, inclusive communities, access to public accommodations) from the various sections of the ADA. Yet, the theme of unfulfilled promise continues with this law as well. Despite assurances in the law banning discrimination in employment against disabled people, the unemployment rate for this community has remained stubbornly high. The proportion of individuals with intellectual or developmental disabilities participating in integrated employment had actually dropped to about 20% by 2010 (Butterworth et al, 2012, 8). Unemployment and segregated workshops and day programmes still dominate the vocational services offered (Mank, 2007). Finally, in 1999, the Supreme Court culminated two decades of deinstitutionalisation decisions in various lower courts by ruling in the *Olmstead* case (*Olmstead v. L.C.*, 1999) that the ADA legislation from 1990 established that 'unjustified segregation of persons with disabilities constitutes discrimination' (United States Department of Justice, Civil Rights Division, nd). Any institutional setting, the Court found, 'severely diminishes the everyday life activity of individuals'.

However, following the pattern of the earlier legislation, the language of *Olmstead* was full of conditional terms. Segregation was not outlawed as such, but only 'unjustified' segregation. Community-based programmes were required if deemed 'appropriate' by professionals. As a result, again, the promise has led to dramatic movement from institution to community, but left thousands behind, languishing in the remaining public institutions. The population of large, public institutions for people with intellectual disabilities crested in the USA in 1967 (two years before Ian was born), at almost 200,000 people (Scott et al, 2008, 402). By 1997, that number had decreased by over 50% to just fewer than 95,000 (Scott et al, 2008, 402). Today, it is down to just under 30,000 (Larson et al, 2017). In January 1991, New Hampshire became the first state since 1848 to operate no large public institutions (of 16 or more residents) as part of its service system for intellectually and developmentally disabled individuals. Some 14 states have now closed all of their large public institutions (Larson et al, 2017). At the same time the waiting list for small community-based residential arrangements remains desperately high. Delays in placement, compounded by underfunding of programmes and constant threats of further cuts, have left many individuals stranded in the homes of their ageing parents. The Medicaid programme (a national health care system that is jointly funded by state and national governments and is the primary public support programme for residential care of people with developmental disabilities) continued to grow. By 1996, the federal government was spending more on community programmes than it was on institutions. However, the nation was still spending almost $8 billion annually on large congregate care facilities (Braddock et al, 1998, 32).

Conclusion

In the view of historian Daniel Fischer (1977), periods of history can be usefully summarised in one of three categories: evolutionary change; revolutionary change; and involutionary change. Revolutionary change is the relatively rare occasion when something dramatic and often cataclysmic happens (wars, scientific discoveries, etc) that relatively quickly produces a monumental shift in people's lives and experiences. In retrospect, the legislative and judicial achievements for people with intellectual disabilities made in the last decades of the 1900s can seem almost revolutionary in nature. Comparing Emma Wolverton's life with those in the generation that came of age in the 1990s reveals dramatic improvements in the rights and protections accorded to most in the disability community. Compared to others in many parts of the Global South, the lives of most disabled Americans seem undeniably privileged and bountiful. Still, the differences between the promises and the reality remain stark. The changes often seem involutionary in nature rather than revolutionary, a situation where things simply become 'more elaborately the same' (Fischer, 1977, 101) leaving the underlying inequities covered with a veneer of rhetoric and legislation but little substantive progress. In too many cases, almost two decades into the twenty-first century, the stories remain unfinished, just more elaborately told.

References

Braddock, D., Hemp, R., Parish, S., Westrich, J. and Park, H. (1998) 'The state of the states in developmental disabilities: summary of the study', in D. Braddock, R. Hemp, S. Parish and J. Westrich (eds) *The state of the states in developmental disabilities*, Washington, DC: The American Association on Mental Retardation, pp 23–53.

Buck, P. (1950) *The child who never grew*, New York, NY: John Day.

Butterworth, J., Smith, F.A., Hall, A.C., Migliore, A., Winsor, J., Domin, D. and Timmons, J.C. (2012) *StateData: The national report on employment services and outcomes*, Boston, MA: University of Massachusetts, Institute for Community Inclusion.

Carey, A. (2009) *On the margins of citizenship: Intellectual disability and civil rights in twentieth-century America*, Philadelphia, PA: Temple University Press.

Davies, S.P. (1930) *Social control of the mentally deficient*, New York, NY: Thomas Y. Crowell.

Ferguson, P.M. (2008) 'The doubting dance: contributions to a history of parent/professional interactions in early 20th century America', *Research and Practice for Persons with Severe Disabilities*, 33(1–2): 48–58.

Fischer, D.H. (1977) *Growing old in America: The Bland-Lee lectures delivered at Clark University*, New York, NY: Oxford University Press.

Goddard, H.H. (1912) *The Kallikak family*, New York, NY: MacMillan.

Goddard, H.H. (1911) 'Four hundred feeble-minded children classified by the Binet method', *Journal of Psycho-Asthenics*, 15(1/2): 17–30.

Koehler-Pentacoff, E. (2016) *The missing Kennedy: Rosemary Kennedy and the secret bonds of four women*, Baltimore, MD: Bancroft Press.

Kuhlmann, F. (1911) 'Binet and Simon's system for measuring the intelligence of children', *Journal of Psycho-Asthenics*, 15(3/4): 76–92, with 6 plates.

Larson, K.C. (2015) *Rosemary: The hidden Kennedy daughter*, Boston, MA: Houghton Mifflin Harcourt.

Larson, S.A., Eschenbacher, J.J., Anderson, L.L., Taylor, B., Pettingill, S., Hewitt, A., Sowers, M. and Bourne, M.L. (2017) *In-home and residential long-term supports and services for persons with intellectual or developmental disabilities: Status and trends, 2015*, Minneapolis, MN: University of Minnesota, Research and Training Center on Community Living, Institute on Community Integration.

Mank, D. (2007) 'Employment', in S.L. Odom, R.H. Horner, M.E. Snell and J. Blacher (eds), *Handbook of developmental disabilities*, New York, NY: Guilford Press, pp 390–409.

Osgood, R.L. (2008) *The history of special education: A struggle for equality in American public schools*, Westport, CT: Praeger.

Rafter, N.H. (1988) *White trash: The eugenic family studies, 1877–1919*, Boston, MA: Northeastern University Press.

Reeves, H.T. (1938) 'The later years of a noted mental defective', *American Journal on Mental Deficiency*, 43(1): 194–200.

Reilly, P.R. (1991) *The surgical solution: A history of involuntary sterilization in the United States*, Baltimore, MD: The Johns Hopkins University Press.

Rogers, D.E. (1953) *Angel unaware*, Westwood, NJ: Revell.

Scott, N., Lakin, K.C. and Larson, S.A. (2008) 'The 40th anniversary of deinstitutionalization in the United States: Decreasing state institutional populations, 1967–2007', *Intellectual and Developmental Disabilities*, 46(5): 402–5.

Shorter, E. (2000) *The Kennedy family and the story of mental retardation*, Philadelphia, PA: Temple University Press.

Smith, J.D. and Wehmeyer, M.L. (2012) *Good blood; bad blood: Science, nature, and the myth of the Kallikaks*, Washington DC: American Association on Intellectual and Developmental Disabilities.

Straney, S.G. (1994) '*The Kallikak Family:* A genealogical examination of a classic in psychology', *The American Genealogist*, 69(2): 65–80.

Trent, J.W. (1994) *Inventing the feeble mind: A history of mental retardation in the United States*, Berkeley, CA: University of California Press.

United States Census Bureau (1906) *Special reports: Insane and feeble-minded in hospitals and institutions, 1904*, Washington, DC: Government Printing Office.

United States Census Bureau (1943) *16th census of the United States: 1940: Special report on the institutional population 14 years and over*, Washington, DC: Government Printing Office.

United States Department of Justice, Civil Rights Division (nd), https://www.ada.gov/olmstead/olmstead_about.htm

Wallin, J.E.W. (1924) *The education of handicapped children*, Boston, MA: Houghton Mifflin Company.

Wolfensberger, W. (1972) *The principle of normalization in human services*, Toronto: National Institute on Mental Retardation.

Zenderland, L. (1998) *Measuring minds: Henry Herbert Goddard and the origins of American intelligence testing*, New York, NY: Cambridge University Press.

Index

Printed and bound by CPI Group (UK) Ltd, Croydon, CR0 4YY

17/04/2025

14658885-0001

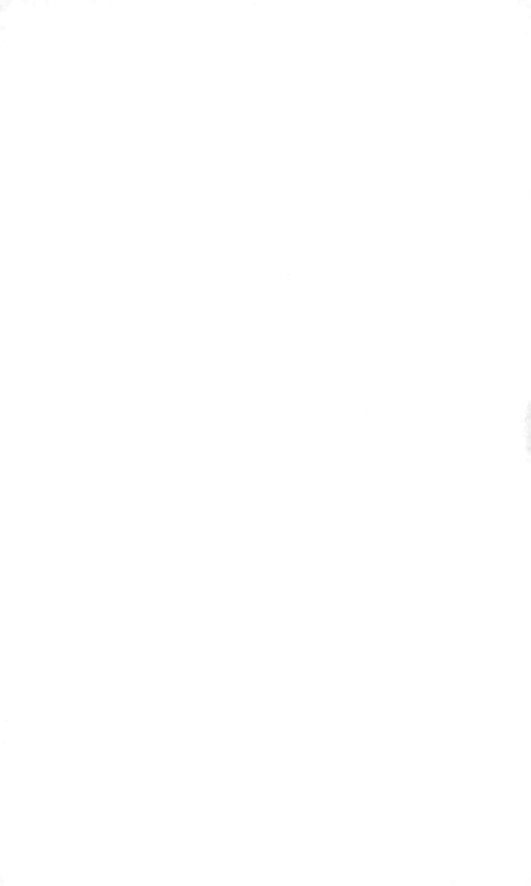